Speech Practice Material

From Sounds to Dialogues

Speech Practice Material
From Sounds to Dialogues

Jack E. Thomas

PLURAL PUBLISHING
INC.
SAN DIEGO
OXFORD
BRISBANE

PLURAL PUBLISHING
INC.

5521 Ruffin Road
San Diego, CA 92123

e-mail: info@pluralpublishing.com
Web site: http://www.pluralpublishing.com

49 Bath Street
Abingdon, Oxfordshire OX14 1EA
United Kingdom

Typeset in 11½/14 Garamond by Flanagan's Publishing Services, Inc.
Printed in the United States of America by McNaughton and Gunn, Inc.
Cover background design by Loren J. Thomas

Library of Congress Cataloging-in-Publication Data

Thomas, Jack E.
Speech practice material : from sounds to dialogues / Jack E. Thomas.
p. ; cm.
Rev. ed. of: Speech practice manual for dysarthria, apraxia, and other disorders of articulation / Robert L. Keith, Jack E. Thomas. 1989.
Includes bibliographical references and index.
ISBN-13: 978-1-59756-287-4 (alk. paper)
ISBN-10: 1-59756-287-4 (alk. paper)
1. Articulation disorders—Treatment. 2. Speech therapy. I. Keith, Robert L. Speech practice manual for dysarthria, apraxia, and other disorders of articulation. II. Title.
[DNLM: 1. Speech Therapy—methods. 2. Speech Disorders—therapy. WL 340.2 T458s 2008]
RC424.7.T46 2008
616.85'506—dc22

2008029350

Contents

Foreword

Clinicians and clinical researchers who work with people who have speech and language disorders face several challenges. Evaluation requires that they select and administer appropriate tasks and tests, and then carefully observe performance. Diagnosis requires a fundamental understanding of numerous speech and language disorders and conclusions that best capture the problem(s) at hand. Along the way, clinicians must estimate severity of the problem and establish the level or levels of the speech system at which the problem resides. A judgment and recommendation must then be made about whether or not therapy will be of benefit, based on clinical experience and available research evidence. If treatment is recommended, then a plan for its focus must be formulated. The clinician must explain what therapy will entail and, if the focus is to improve speech, that it will require hard work, often drill work. At this point, the clinician's position is like that of a builder who has a contract and the plans for a house in hand, but no materials with which to build it. This position is no less true for the clinical researcher who must develop tasks for a new treatment, or tasks for testing hypotheses about the nature of disordered speech.

In *Speech Practice Material: From Sounds to Dialogues*, Jack Thomas provides the materials for building treatment or clinical research tasks for a wide variety of speech problems. There is a wealth of materials here—more than needed for any single patient or speech disorder. They range from nuts and bolts (sounds and words) to major arches and frames (common expressions, figurative language, dialogues). Users of this manual should know that it has been developed by an outstanding, expert clinician who has treated a wide variety of communication disorders long enough to know what stands the test of time. This manual is a well-stocked toolbox, one assembled by a clinician for clinicians and clinical researchers. Keep it handy. Use it wisely.

Joseph R. Duffy, Ph.D

Preface

The first edition of this book was entitled, *Speech Practice Manual for Dysarthria, Apraxia and Other Disorders of Articulation: Compare and Contrast*. I wrote it with my colleague, friend, mentor, and expert clinician, Robert (Bob) L. Keith. Published in 1989, it was a collection of practice materials we had developed independently, with many of them created by Bob during his 32 years of experience treating patients with neurogenic speech and language disorders, as well as patients with head and neck cancer. It is due in large part to Robert Keith's tutelage and his method of developing therapy materials, that is, listen to the patient, create what he or she needs, modify it as you go along, keep it for the next similar patient, that I learned to develop therapy materials for my patients, as well as to study the literature and weigh the evidence for applying particular treatments or stimuli.

At about the same time I started to revise the book on my own, I attended a speech-language pathology seminar to learn about a particular treatment technique. It was grounded in sound theory and has been proven to be effective in well-controlled studies. Despite such respectable outcomes, I was concerned by the inflexibility of the treatment protocol and stimuli. Afterward, when I met with my next new patient who fit the criteria for that treatment, my concerns were reinforced. The specific treatment protocol didn't fit him—his life, his predicament, his "big picture." With little or no room for strategic modification, this and other treatments with evidence supporting their efficacy don't fit many patients for whom they are intended. As Frattali and Worrall (2001, p. ix) remind us, "Not even the best of large-scale or randomized clinical trials can take the place of well-sharpened clinical judgment, made on a patient-by-patient basis."

The speech materials in this book are not based on or related to any particular treatment program. They are intended to be versatile, flexible, and used in many ways for many populations. Some of the stimuli are tried-and-true with some new variations. Others are unique. Some particular therapy techniques and variations on how to use and alter the material are suggested in this book, but no particular theory or step-by-step approach is recommended or supported. Decisions about whom to use it with, how, and why, are in the hands, judgment, and creativity of the clinician. The expectation is that modifications of all material and any procedure will be necessary for most clients.

The contents of this book are organized in a similar manner across most of the chapters. First, the therapy materials are described and examples are provided. Next, the populations for which the material might be used, referred to as "Disorder-Specific Applications," are suggested. For example, the scripted conversations that appear in Chapter 8, Dialogues, may have application, depending on the severity of the problem, to apraxia of speech, dysarthria, speech after laryngectomy or glossectomy, or other head and neck cancer surgeries and treatments, voice disorders, stuttering, pragmatic communication skills, social and regional dialects, foreign accent modification, and American English as a second language. The next section contains a table of possible Goal Areas (e.g., articulation/phonology, rate, prosody) and corresponding Target Skills (e.g., specific phonemes, reduced speaking rate, customary intonational-prosodic patterns for statements, questions, and exclamations). Suggestions are presented for implementing and modifying the stimuli for any given client. This is followed by the stimuli, which are consistently presented in a shorter-to-longer, simple-to-more complex order. At the end of most chapters is a form to assist individualizing practice material for each client.

Chapter 1, Automatic Speech Tasks, presents seriatim speech and overlearned sequences of words that can be used with different client populations.

Chapter 2, Consonants, and Chapter 3, Vowels and Diphthongs, contain hundreds of minimal pairs and other sound contrasts in real words. These are followed by two-word phrases containing the target sound, two-word phrases containing the target sound and a variety of contrasted sounds, and then sentences with the target and contrasts.

Chapter 4, Word Grids, contains most consonants, consonant clusters, vowels, and diphthongs in short words for typical and unique comparisons of sounds at a glance.

Chapter 5, Common Expressions, includes many common greetings, comments, responses, questions, retorts, and exclamations frequently used in everyday conversations.

Chapter 6, Figurative Expressions, features figurative language of many types—idioms, proverbs, clichés, and other abstract forms—which are used in everyday conversation.

Chapter 7, Speaking with Exaggerated Articulatory Movements, is intended for some clients who do not open their mouths sufficiently when they speak and/or their articulation is imprecise and intelligibility is reduced. The sentence stimuli are for practice of over-articulation.

Chapter 8, Dialogues, presents scripted conversations between two people. They are light, familiar, and humorous dialogues for practicing a wide variety of speech skills, such as conversational turn-taking, prosodic variations, timing and rhythm, tone of voice, specific speech sounds, fluency, and common and figurative expressions.

Chapter 9, Contrastive Stress Drills, reviews the therapy technique of contrastive stress drill and how it brings conversational prosody into the drill and practice associated with management of speech-sound disorders.

Chapter 10, Keeping on Track with Base-10 Response Forms, presents and describes the Base-10 Response Form as a convenient way to organize speech therapy tasks, keep data, and analyze client performance.

Again, there are no rules for using these materials. Only one strong and obvious recommendation can be given—think critically! Study and apply the best evidence and practice guidelines from the current professional literature. Confer with experienced colleagues. Do what best suits the client's needs and fits his or her "big picture" needs.

Jack E. Thomas

Acknowledgments

Special thanks to all the patients who served as my teachers, and to Robert L. Keith for his guidance, mentoring, and friendship.

There are a few texts that I have found particularly valuable and necessary for learning about neurogenic speech disorders and how to intervene to reduce their impact.

Motor Speech Disorders: Substrates, Differential Diagnosis, and Management, Second Edition (2005), by Joseph R. Duffy is an invaluable scholarly and practical work, packed with clear thinking and science, and brimming with information for diagnosis and treatment in everyday practice. Well organized, comprehensive, and remarkably detailed, it is indispensable to even the most experienced and knowledgeable medical speech-language pathologist.

Apraxia of Speech in Adults: The Disorder and Its Management (1991) by Wertz, LaPointe, and Rosenbek, three of the profession's finest scientists, clinicians, and teachers, provides excellent guidance and critical thinking and should be at the fingertips of all speech-language pathologists working with apraxia of speech.

Management of Motor Speech Disorders in Children and Adults, Second Edition (1999), by Yorkston, Beukelman, Strand, and Bell, is an outstanding resource, presenting descriptions of various neurologic communication disorders and treatments for them that are organized into stages and lead to sensible clinical decisions that vary depending on the level of the client's functional limitations.

I think of these authors as my colleagues and mentors, helping me and fellow speech-language pathologists become the best clinicians we can be, not only with neurogenic patient populations, but with others as well. They have my deepest and heartfelt thanks and appreciation.

To
Linda and Loren

1

Automatic Speech Tasks

Some clients show us and others tell us that certain words are easier for them to say than others. This is the case with some patients with acquired neurologic communication disorders of apraxia of speech, dysarthria, and aphasia. Darley (1982, p. 11) stated "Apraxic patients display a marked discrepancy between their relatively good performance on automatic and reactive speech productions and their relatively poor volitional-purposive speech performance." He quoted Schuell, Jenkins, and Jimenez-Pabon (1964) who wrote about patients with apraxia of speech, "Words and phrases highly organized by practice and usage tend to sound normal." Other clients agree, including some with dysarthria, those who stutter, people with certain voice disorders, and those with aphasic language disturbance. Often the easier words are seriatim words we practiced over and over when we were children, such as counting, the alphabet, the days of the week, and others. Simple rhymes and songs from childhood may also fall into this "automatic" category. Obviously, counting out loud and singing "Happy Birthday" have limited usefulness for communication in most people's lives. Yet, practicing relatively easy automatic and overlearned series of words can be worthwhile in speech-language therapy. Using automatic speech can permit the speaker to direct cognitive resources toward the motor planning and execution of speech elements rather than to the purposive, communicative content of most verbal language.

How can automatic speech be used in therapy and with what populations?

DISORDER-SPECIFIC APPLICATIONS

Apraxia of Speech and Dysarthria

For people with apraxia of speech or dysarthria, the automatic speech material in this section may be used to work on articulation, timing/rhythm, melody, loudness, and rate. For some people with severe apraxia of speech or dysarthria, these stimuli and material like them may help to promote basic phonation and the simplest of speech movements. If language or other cognitive impairment is present, which is often the case in these populations, the printed stimuli may help the client stay on task, and they provide graphemic cues that may facilitate improved speech performance.

Voice Disorders

For people with hyperfunctional voice disorders who have achieved approximated or target voice production in vowel prolongation and short utterances, practicing the desired voice in these most familiar words and phrases may be an early step in the continuum of therapy stimuli. Subsequent steps may include the more purposive, conversational speech practice material found in Common Expressions (Chapter 5), Figurative Expressions (Chapter 6), and Dialogues (Chapter 8).

Laryngectomy

For people who have had a total laryngectomy who use an artificial larynx device, a tracheoesophageal voice prosthesis, or use esophageal voice, and for those who have had any of the wide variety of other laryngeal surgeries, the material in this section may be helpful for pairing breathing and phrasing, pacing, as well as for addressing pitch, loudness, and voice quality.

Glossectomy and Other Head and Neck Cancer Surgeries and Treatments

For people who have had partial or total glossectomy, other head and neck surgeries, and/or chemoradiation treatments to the head and neck that compromise articulatory precision, this material may be used to explore and practice compensatory articulatory gestures, to practice speaking at a reduced rate, and to experiment with pitch and prosodic variations to enhance intelligibility.

Dialects of American English

For people wishing to reduce their specific social or regional dialect, this material may be used to address production of all speech sounds and syllables in common words in mainstream American English.

Foreign Accent Modification and English as a Second Language

For people wishing to reduce their foreign accent and for those learning American English as a second language, this material, particularly counting, days of the week, and other word series, is valuable for learning fundamental words in American English, to practice specific speech sounds, to learn stress and durational elements in polysyllabic words, to study sound-symbol association with some of the first words encountered in learning English as second language, and to practice a speaking rate that maximizes intelligibility.

EXAMPLES OF GOAL AREAS AND TARGET SKILLS THAT CAN BE ADDRESSED BY AUTOMATIC SPEECH TASKS

Goal Areas	Target Skills
Articulation/Phonology	• producing basic speech sounds and movements in the most common and automatic words of American English • specific phonemes in various word positions • consonant clusters and sound blending • polysyllabic words • overall intelligibility
Rate	• reduced speaking rate • increased speaking rate
Prosody	• variable pitch • variable loudness • prosody and timing in automatic and seriatim speech of American English • conventional stress patterns of common polysyllabic words • prolongation of vowels and appropriate consonants to practice motor speech control • syllable-by-syllable approach to speaking • breath control; manner of breathing • phrasing
Fluency	• using a prolonged-speech technique for fluent production of specific sounds, frequently used words, and phrases • coordinating breathing and phrasing • naturalness
Voice	• consistent phonation • increased loudness • decreased loudness • best possible voice (free of hoarseness, breathiness, and roughness with appropriate pitch and loudness) • breath support; manner of breathing • phrasing

Conversational Skills	• underlying speech skills for maximal intelligibility in conversation
Social or Regional Dialect Modification	• articulation of specific speech sounds that are habitually omitted, substituted, or distorted • inclusion of all syllables of words • stress patterns and other prosodic elements of polysyllabic words in mainstream American English
Foreign Accent Reduction and American English as a Second Language	• common, frequently used words in American English • articulation of specific sounds in American English that are habitually omitted, substituted, or distorted • inclusion of all syllables of words • stress patterns and other prosodic elements of polysyllabic words in American English • intonational-prosodic patterns of American English • slower speaking rate to maximize intelligibility

SUGGESTIONS FOR USING AND MODIFYING THE SPEECH PRACTICE MATERIAL IN AUTOMATIC SPEECH TASKS

- Use highlighting, underlining, arrows, slashes, and other diacritical markings to indicate the presence of specific speech sounds, to emphasize them, to indicate pauses or where to breathe, alteration in rate, prolongation, changes in loudness, pitch-prosodic variation, and so forth.
- Address one of the client's speech goals—such as prolongation of vowels and diphthongs—during one practice session, then switch to another of the patient's goals, such as "naturalness" during a subsequent practice of the same material. Later, address both goals simultaneously.
- In everyday circumstances, seriatim speech is usually spoken quite rapidly. However, depending on the client and the goal of the exercise, the clinician may want the client to practice slow, contemplative production of these words to facilitate accurate articulation, syllable-by-syllable production, and so forth. Throughout the therapy session consider demonstrating a deliberate, slower than normal pace as a model for the client, exaggerating and emphasizing the aspects of speech that are the client's actual therapy targets.
- Self-monitoring and thinking about one's performance are an essential part of the process for improving speech and language skills. A tried-and-true therapy procedure is to audio-or-video record the client pro-

ducing automatic speech, then review the recordings with the client to analyze the speech performance.

- The material in Automatic Speech Tasks can be altered easily to reduce its rote or automatic character. Examples: Practice sequences of words such as counting, the days of the week, and the months of the year in reverse order. Link two stimulus items together with the word "and" or "or," such as "one and two; three and four"; "January or February; March or April." Link other material in this section such as Common Opposites and Words That Go Together, such as "up and down and yes and no"; "bacon and eggs and salt and pepper." Remove the printed words and provide the client with only one of the words of a pair, such as, "Black" and expect a response of "and white." Reverse common word pairs, such as "west and east" and "meatballs and spaghetti." Use the question-response format of Contrastive Stress Drills (Chapter 9) with the material in Automatic Speech Tasks, such as, Question: "Bacon and *spaghetti*?" Response: "No, bacon and *eggs*."
- Delete or change practice material that distract the client from the goals of therapy.

PRACTICE MATERIALS FOR AUTOMATIC SPEECH TASKS

Counting (numbers spelled out)

one	two	three
four	five	six
seven	eight	nine
ten	eleven	twelve
thirteen	fourteen	fifteen
sixteen	seventeen	eighteen
nineteen	twenty	twenty-one
twenty-two	twenty-three	twenty-four
twenty-five	twenty-six	twenty-seven
twenty-eight	twenty-nine	thirty
thirty-one	thirty-two	thirty-three
thirty-four	thirty-five	thirty-six
thirty-seven	thirty-eight	thirty-nine
forty	forty-one	forty-two
forty-three	forty-four	forty-five
forty-six	forty-seven	forty-eight
forty-nine	fifty	fifty-one
fifty-two	fifty-three	fifty-four
fifty-five	fifty-six	fifty-seven
fifty-eight	fifty-nine	sixty
sixty-one	sixty-two	sixty-three
sixty-four	sixty-five	sixty-six
sixty-seven	sixty-eight	sixty-nine
seventy	seventy-one	seventy-two
seventy-three	seventy-four	seventy-five
seventy-six	seventy-seven	seventy-eight
seventy-nine	eighty	eighty-one
eighty-two	eighty-three	eighty-four

eighty-five	eighty-six	eighty-seven
eighty-eight	eighty-nine	ninety
ninety-one	ninety-two	ninety-three
ninety-four	ninety-five	ninety-six
ninety-seven	ninety-eight	ninety-nine
one hundred	one hundred one	one hundred two
one hundred three	one hundred four	one hundred five
one hundred six	one hundred seven	one hundred eight
one hundred nine	one hundred ten	one hundred eleven
one hundred twelve	one hundred thirteen	one hundred fourteen
one hundred fifteen	one hundred sixteen	one hundred seventeen

Counting

1	2	3	4	5
6	7	8	9	10
11	12	13	14	15
16	17	18	19	20
21	22	23	24	25
26	27	28	29	30
31	32	33	34	35
36	37	38	39	40
41	42	43	44	45
46	47	48	49	50
51	52	53	54	55
56	57	58	59	60
61	62	63	64	65
66	67	68	69	70
71	72	73	74	75
76	77	78	79	80
81	82	83	84	85
86	87	88	89	90
91	92	93	94	95
96	97	98	99	100

Counting by 10s

10	20	30	40	50
60	70	80	90	100
110	120	130	140	150
160	170	180	190	200
210	220	230	240	250
260	270	280	290	300
310	320	330	340	350
360	370	380	390	400
410	420	430	440	450
460	470	480	490	500

Counting by 5s

5	10	15	20	25
30	35	40	45	50
55	60	65	70	75
80	85	90	95	100
105	110	115	120	125
130	135	140	145	150
155	160	165	170	175
180	185	190	195	200

Alphabet

A	B	C	D	E
F	G	H	I	J
K	L	M	N	O
P	Q	R	S	T
U	V	W	X	Y
Z				

Vowels

A	E	I	O	U

Days of the Week

Sunday	Monday	Tuesday	Wednesday
Thursday	Friday	Saturday	

Months of the Year

January	February	March	April
May	June	July	August
September	October	November	December

Time (words written out)

one o'clock	two o'clock	three o'clock	four o'clock
five o'clock	six o'clock	seven o'clock	eight o'clock
nine o'clock	ten o'clock	eleven o'clock	twelve o'clock

Time (hour, quarter hour, half hour, three-quarter hour)

1:00	2:00	3:00	4:00
5:00	6:00	7:00	8:00
9:00	10:00	11:00	12:00
1:15	2:15	3:15	4:15
5:15	6:15	7:15	8:15
9:15	10:15	11:15	12:15
1:30	2:30	3:30	4:30
5:30	6:30	7:30	8:30
9:30	10:30	11:30	12:30
1:45	2:45	3:45	4:45
5:45	6:45	7:45	8:45
9:45	10:45	11:45	12:45

Time (AM and PM)

1 AM	2 AM	3 AM	4 AM
5 AM	6 AM	7 AM	8 AM
9 AM	10 AM	11 AM	12 PM
1:30 PM	2:30 PM	3:30 PM	4:30 PM
5:30 PM	6:30 PM	7:30 PM	8:30 PM
9:30 PM	10:30 PM	11:30 PM	12:30 AM

Common Opposites

up - down	yes - no
stop - go	in - out
good - bad	men - women
north - south	young - old
boys - girls	near - far
on - off	night - day
hard - soft	hot - cold
left - right	high - low
early - late	front - back
sweet - sour	wet - dry
open - shut	true - false
laugh - cry	war - peace
lost - found	east - west
black - white	quiet - loud
summer - winter	over - under
tall - short	weak - strong
add - subtract	brother - sister

Words That Go Together

bacon and eggs	salt and pepper
pots and pans	nickels and dimes
hammer and nails	dogs and cats
shoes and socks	now and then
bread and butter	knife and fork
meat and potatoes	hands and feet
arms and legs	peanut butter and jelly
table and chairs	spaghetti and meatballs
soap and water	stars and stripes
cats and dogs	soup and sandwich
cake and ice cream	crackers and cheese
mashed potatoes and gravy	hamburger and French fries

Other Sources of Automatic Speech:

- Nursery rhymes
- Prayers
- Slogans and mottos
- Organization and club pledges
- Songs/chants

2

Consonants

This practice material was designed to provide many opportunities to practice production of specific consonants in fairly common words, and in phrases and sentences, all with emphasis of comparing the target speech sound in minimal pairs and other contrasting environments.

The author's introduction to minimal contrasts was in Fairbanks' *Voice and Articulation Drillbook* (1960). Fairbanks' method of " . . . work toward the sound in question from a similar sound" (p. 27), and comparing words differing by only one element, is an obvious and natural way to approach speech-sound disorders in both children and adults. Later, Weiner (1981) described a phonologic treatment approach—a variation of a procedure by Cooper (1968)—using meaningful contrastive minimal pairs that was successful for some children with severe speech-sound disorders. Since then, treating children with phonological disorders has evolved in a number of directions, with many of them moving beyond minimal pairs contrasts to incorporating various other speech sound contrasts (Kamhi & Pollock, 2005). Yet, the technique of comparing and contrasting phonemes in CVC words to remediate speech-sound disorders continues for both children and adults. For example, there is evidence that minimal contrast practice, used along with other techniques such as integral stimulation, articulatory placement cuing, and presentation of graphic cues is " . . . likely to provide gains in speech production for individuals with apraxia of speech even when deficits are chronic and severe" (Wambaugh, Duffy, McNeil, Robin, & Rogers, 2006, pp. xlvii–xlviii).

In the speech practice material presented here, most consonants in American English are represented in the initial and final positions of short words. Most common consonant clusters are represented in the initial position of short words. The following table provides examples of how the material is arranged for each consonant, starting with consonant-vowel-consonant (CVC) words, then to phrases, polysyllabic words, and sentences with multiple speech sound contrasts and with the target consonant appearing in all word positions. Throughout these materials a broad phonemic transcription is applied. Some speech sounds are grouped in nontraditional ways.

DESCRIPTION AND EXAMPLES OF PRACTICE MATERIAL IN THIS CHAPTER

Description of Practice Material for Consonants	Examples of Practice Material for /b/
Target consonant in the initial position of CVC words with most vowels and diphthongs represented	beach, bead, beef bib, big, bill babe, bake, base
Target consonant in the initial position of CVC words in two-word phrases	book bag bed bug bang-bang
Target consonant in the final position of CVC words	bib, fib, rib dab, gab, jab gob, job, sob
Target consonant in the final position of both CVC words in two-word phrases	cob web lube job rob Abe
Target consonant in the initial position of the first word and in the final position of the second word in two-word phrases	big fib bad curb ball club
Target consonant in the initial position of CVC words and contrasted in minimal pairs	beach - peach; big - pig; bet - pet buck - duck; ball - doll; bark - dark base - vase; ban - van; boat - vote
Target consonant in the initial position of the first CVC word in two-word phrases with the second word beginning with a contrasting consonant	bake pie, bean pod, back pain boat dock, big ditch, burn down ball mitt, big map, bad mood
Target consonant plus consonant (cluster) in the initial position of short words	bleach, bleed, bleak brew, broom, bruise
Target consonant in the initial position of words of increasing length and phrases	bare, barefoot, barefooted base, baseball, baseball park bathe, bathing, bathing suit
Target consonant in all positions of words in sentences that contain multiple contrasts to the target	Get that big cobweb. Polly bought a new bowling ball. I'm a big fan of barbecue beef. My neighbors bought a new boat. Pat's homemade blackberry pie is the best.

How can practice material for specific consonants be used in therapy and with what populations? Suggestions follow, but obviously, the clinician must determine the appropriateness of practice material for any given client, weighing the type and severity of the speech disorder, and the client's capabilities.

DISORDER-SPECIFIC APPLICATIONS

Apraxia of Speech

For people with apraxia of speech, this section includes many minimal pair contrasts and other consonant oppositions in short words and phrases for drill on articulatory precision, prosodic naturalness, and for modifying temporal dimensions. These precede sentence-length material containing the same consonant targets with various oppositions.

In adults, aphasic language impairment usually accompanies apraxia of speech. Some of the material in this book intended to address various phonologic impairments, motor speech disorders, and other disorders of speech production may also be applicable to a given client's language impairment.

Dysarthria

For people with dysarthria, speech practice material juxtaposing consonants in short words, phrases, and sentences may be suitable for therapy goals similar to those for treating apraxia of speech, including articulatory precision, elements of prosody, speaking rate, a syllable-by-syllable approach to speaking, and loudness.

Laryngectomy

For people who have had a total laryngectomy who use an artificial larynx device, tracheoesophageal voice prosthesis, or esophageal voice, and for those who have had other laryngeal surgeries to ablate disease, this speech practice material may be helpful for improving articulation, increasing oral openness when speaking, coordinating breathing with voice production, phrasing, pacing-timing, as well as for addressing loudness and voice quality.

Glossectomy and Other Head and Neck Cancer Surgeries and Treatments

For people who have had partial or total glossectomy, other head and neck surgeries, and/or chemoradiation treatments to the head and neck that compromise articulatory precision and/or voice, this material may be used to explore and practice compensatory articulatory gestures, and to practice speaking at a reduced rate.

Modifying Social or Regional Dialects of American English

For people wishing to modify their specific social or regional dialect, this material may be utilized to differentiate and practice consonant sounds of American English that are habitually omitted, substituted, or distorted. In addition, customary grammatical structure of American English may be practiced in the phrase-length and sentence-length material.

Foreign Accent Modification and Learning American English as a Second Language

For people wishing to reduce their foreign accent and for those learning American English as a second language, this material will provide many pages of speech practice material that focus on all consonant sounds in common words in American English, and common and predictable articulatory substitutions of speakers of particular languages by contrasting the target sounds with their habitual substitutions in CVC words, and in phrases and sentences. In addition, the material in other sections of the book are appropriate to practice an optimal speaking rate (usually a reduced rate), to maximize intelligibility, to focus on customary stress and prosodic patterns of polysyllabic words and various sentence types, and to learn timing and other pragmatic-social aspects of American English conversation.

EXAMPLES OF GOAL AREAS AND TARGET SKILLS THAT CAN BE ADDRESSED BY MATERIAL IN THIS CHAPTER

Goal Areas	Target Skills
Phonology/Articulation	• articulation of specific consonants • juxtaposing similar speech sounds in simple and more complex linguistic environments • overall intelligibility
Rate	• reduce speaking rate • increase speaking rate • intelligibility • naturalness
Prosody	• conventional intonational-prosodic patterns in phrases and sentences • syllable-by-syllable production of words, phrases, and sentences • pitch and loudness variations • manner of breathing; breath control • phrasing • fluency and smoothness • naturalness
Fluency	• using a prolonged-speech technique to produce specific sounds, words, phrases, and sentences • naturalness

Voice	• best possible voice quality (free of hoarseness, breathiness, roughness, with appropriate pitch) • increased loudness • reduced loudness • breath support; manner of breathing • phrasing
Social or Regional Dialect Modification	• articulation of specific consonants that are habitually omitted, substituted, or distorted • inclusion of all syllables in words and sentences in American English • conventional prosodic patterns of mainstream American English • intelligibility
Foreign Accent Reduction and American English as a Second Language	• slower speaking rate to maximize intelligibility • articulation of specific consonants of American English that are habitually substituted, distorted, or omitted • inclusion of all syllables of words in sentences • conventional intonational-stress-prosodic patterns of mainstream American English • intelligibility • naturalness

SUGGESTIONS FOR USING AND MODIFYING THE PRACTICE MATERIAL IN THIS CHAPTER

- Use highlighting, underlining, arrows, slashes, and other diacritical markings to indicate the presence of specific consonant sounds, to stress/emphasize them, to indicate pauses, alteration in rate, prolongation, change in loudness, pitch-prosodic variation, and so forth.
- Address one of the client's speech goals, such as articulatory precision, then during subsequent practice of the same material, switch to another of the client's goals, such as naturalness. Later, address both goals simultaneously.
- Depending on specific goals, the clinician may choose to demonstrate to the client a deliberate, slower than normal model to emphasize a particular speech target.
- Self-monitoring and self-critique are fundamental to improving speech skills. A tried-and-true therapy procedure is to audio-record or video-record the client during speech practice. Afterward, the

clinician and client can review the recordings and analyze the speech performance.

- To change the two-word phrases into slightly more complex three-word phrases, add an adjective or pronoun to the noun phrases, such as "*a* big park," "*one* big perch," and "*my* bad putt." Words that can most often precede noun phrases are "a," "the," "one," "this," "that," "my," "his," and "her."
- For additional practice of polysyllabic words beginning with a particular consonant, create phrases or sentences with the words appearing in the "Words of Increasing Length and Phrases" section for that consonant.
- Most of the speech practice material in all sections of this book can be modified or used directly for practice of consonant targets.
- For additional variations of contrasting consonants in simple to more complex linguistic environments, refer to the Word Grids (Chapter 4) and Contrastive Stress Drills (Chapter 9).
- Consider using Base-10 Response Forms (Chapter 10) for organizing treatment and scoring and plotting performance on speech management tasks for consonants.
- Delete or modify speech practice material that distracts the client from the intended goals of therapy.

PRACTICE MATERIAL FOR CONSONANTS

b__

bee, beach, bead, beef, beak, beam, bean, beep, beet, bees
bib, big, bill, bin, bit
bay, babe, bake, bale, base, bait, bathe
bed, beg, bell, Ben, Bess, bet, Beth
batch, bad, bag, badge, back, ban, bass, bash, bat, bath
bud, buff, bug, budge, buck, bum, bun, bus, but, buzz
Bob, botch, bog, ball, bomb, bop, boss, bought
bow, bowl, bone, boat, both, bows
boo, booed, boom, boot, booth
book, bush
butte
bough, bowel, boughs
buy, bike, bite
boy, Boyd, boil, boys
burr, birch, bird, burn, burp, Burt, birth, burrs
beer, beard
bear, bears
bar, Barb, barge, bark, barn, Bart, bars
bore, board, born, bores

b__ b__ Phrases

book bag
big bomb
Big Ben
bed bug
buy beef
bang-bang
bad boys
big boot
bar bell

birch bark
bad back
big book
back bone
bell boy
beach bum
big boat
bad book
bird bath

bug bite
bait box
bean bag
big boom
bad burn
beach ball
bad bet
big bass
brown boots

__b

bib, fib, rib
Abe, babe
Deb, web
dab, gab, jab, cab, lab, nab, tab
dub, hub, cub, rub, sub, tub
Bob, gob, job, cob, mob, knob, rob, sob
lube, tube
lobe, robe
herb, verb
Barb

__b __b Phrases

cob web
lube job
rob Abe

b__ __b Phrases

big fib
bar tab
big mob
big tub
bad curb
big crib
ball club
boil crab
boys' club

b – d Contrasts

bee - Dee
bead - deed
bean - dean
beep - deep

bid - did
big - dig
Bill - dill

bay - day
bale - Dale
bait - date
bays - days

bed - dead
Ben - den
Beth - death

bad - dad
bam - dam
ban - Dan

bash - dash
bud - dud
bug - dug
buck - duck
bum - dumb
bun - done
buzz - does

bog - dog
ball - doll
bought - dot

bow - dough

boo - due
booed - dude
boom - doom

bout - doubt

buy - die
buys -dyes

Bert - dirt
beer - deer

bear - dare

bark - dark
barn - darn
Bart - dart

bore - door

b__ d__ Phrases

boat dock
boot-deep
big ditch
bear den

back down
big deck
back dues
burn down

black dot
black death
beat down
buckle down

b – g Contrasts

bill - gill

babe - Gabe
bail - Gayle
bait - gate
bays - gaze

Bess - guess
bet - get

bass - gas
bash - gash

bum - gum
bun - gun
bus - Gus
but - gut

Bob - gob
bought - got

bow - go
bowl - goal
bows - goes

bout - gout

buy - guy

beer - gear
beard - geared

bored - gourd

b__ g__ Phrases

buy gas
be good
big goat
bad guess

ball game
big goose
back gate
bad guy

ball gown
bad gash
big goof
big gut

b – m Contrasts

be – me
beak – meek
bean – mean
beet – meet

bill – mill
bit – mitt

bay – may
bake – make
bail – mail
base – mace
bait – mate

beg – Meg
bell – Mel
Ben – men
Bess – mess
bet – met

batch – match
bad – mad

badge – Madge
back – Mac
ban – man
bass – mass
bash – mash
bat – mat

bud – mud
bug – mug
buck – muck
bum – mum
bus – muss
but – mutt

baa – ma
Bob – mob
ball – mall
bomb – mom
bop – mop
boss – moss

boo – moo
booed – mood
boot – moot

butte – mute

bow – mow
bowl – mole

bone – moan
boat – moat

by – my
bike – Mike
bite – might

bear – mare

bar – mar
barge – Marge
bark – mark

bore – more

b__ m__ Phrases

be mine
bad meal
ball mitt
big myth
bad men
bath mat

book mark
big mess
Bat Man
big map
big mob
Big Mac

big mouth
big moth
boil meat
bench mark
bad mood
bad move

b – p Contrasts

bee - pea
beach - peach
beak - peak
beep - peep
beat - Pete
bees - peas

big - pig
bill - pill
bin - pin
bit - pit

bale - pale
bays - pays

beg - peg
Ben - pen
bet - pet

batch - patch
bad - pad
back - pack
ban - pan
bass - pass
bat - pat
bath - path

bub - pub
buff - puff
bug - pug
bun - pun
bus - pus
but - putt

ball - Paul
bop - pop

bought - pot

bull - pull

bowel - Powell

buy - pie
bike - pike

birch - perch

bar - par
bark - park
Bart - part

bore - pour

b__ p__ Phrases

bake pie
ball park
boat pier
bird perch
bad part
boil pork
back porch
big pear
back page

big pig
bean pod
big perch
beer pub
berry pie
boil peas
big peak
back pack
bean patch

back pain
bean pot
big park
bear paw
bus pass
bad putt
back pay
bad pun
beach party

b – v Contrasts

Bic - Vic

bale - veil

base - vase

bet - vet

ban - van

bat - vat

boat - vote

bough - vow

burn - Vern

beer - veer

bl__

bleach, bleed, bleak, bleep

blip, bliss

blade, Blake, blame, blaze

bled, bless

blab, black

blood, blush

blob, blotch, block, blot

blow, blows

blue, bloom, blues

blur

blare

br__

breach, breed, breathe, breeze

bridge, brick, brim

braid, break, Braille, brain, brace, brave

bread, breath

Brad, bran, brass, brash, brat

broad, brawl, brawn

brew, brood, broom, brute, bruise

brook

brow, brown

bride, brine, bright

Words of Increasing Length and Phrases That Begin with /b/

bare

bed

base

back

back

batter

bathe

black

beans

barefoot

bedside

baseball

background

back seat

battering

bathing

black strap

baked beans

barefooted

bedside manner

baseball park

background music

back-seat driver

battering ram

bathing suit

black strap molasses

Boston baked beans

Sentences with /b/

1. I'll be back.
2. Get that big cobweb.
3. Park the cab by the curb.
4. Both boys got bad bumps.
5. Bill bought a new bowling ball.
6. The wind blew my birch to bits.
7. My neighbors bought a new boat.
8. Our baseball team beat the Bears.
9. The bass were biting at Big Lake.
10. Put the bird bath in my back yard.
11. Don't burn the banana bread again.
12. Bonnie's blackberry pie is the best.
13. Ben heard sobbing from the bedroom.
14. The big bands will begin to play soon.
15. Bellboy, please put my bag in that cab.
16. "Good night, boys, don't let the bedbugs bite."
17. That book may be a big seller, but it bored me.
18. I'll bet you a buck Pat blows his big date with Beth.
19. Boy, this lemon pie is much better than one you buy at a bakery.
20. "Boogie Woogie Bugle Boy of Company B" was a big hit for Bette Midler.

/tʃ/__

chief, cheek, cheap, cheat, cheese
chick, chill, chin, chip
chafe, chain, chase
check, chess
Chad, chap, chat
chug, Chuck, chum
chalk, chop
choke, chose
chew, chewed, choose
chow
chide, chime, chive
choice
churn, chirp
cheer, cheered
chair
char, charred, charm, chart
chore

tʃ__ tʃ__ Phrases

cheap cheese	choice cheese	chirp-chirp
charred chop	charm Chad	choice chops
choke chain	choose Chuck	chaffed chin
chop-chop	chill cheese	chess champ
cheap chair	chase Chuck	Charlie's cheap

__tʃ

each, beach, leech, peach, reach, teach
itch, ditch, hitch, Mitch, pitch, rich, witch
fetch, wretch
batch, hatch, catch, latch, match, patch, thatch
Dutch, much, such, touch
botch, notch, watch

coach, poach, roach
hooch, mooch, pooch
ouch, couch, pouch, vouch
birch, church, lurch, perch, search
arch, parch
porch, torch

__tʃ __tʃ Phrases

catch perch
teach Mitch
each batch
teach Dutch
speech coach
each stitch
rich grouch

tʃ__ __tʃ Phrases

chess match
check each
cheap batch
choice beach
chess coach
chide Mitch
choice catch
chilled peach
chain stitch

tʃ – k Contrasts

cheap – keep
cheese – keys

chick – kick
chill – kill
chin – kin

chain – cane
chase - case

chap – cap
chat – cat

chub – cub
chum – come

chew – coo
chewed – cooed

choke - Coke

chow – cow

chair – care
chairs – cares

char – car
charred – card
chart – cart

chore – core

tʃ__ k__ Phrases

Chad can
choice corn
chess king
cheap coin
Chuck's cat
China cup
chicken coop
chicken cage
chart a course

tʃ – dʒ Contrasts

cheap – Jeep

chill – Jill
chin – gin

chain – Jane

chess – Jess

chug – jug

choke – joke

cheer – jeer

tʃ – ʃ Contrasts

cheap – sheep
cheat – sheet

chin – shin
chip – ship

chalk – shock
chop – shop

chose – shows

chew – shoe
choose – shoes

cheer – sheer

chair – share

chore – shore

tʃ__ ʃ__ Phrases

cheap shoes
cheese shop

cheap shot
choice sheep

cheap shop
cheap show

tʃ – t Contrasts

cheek – teak
cheese – tease

chick – tick
chill – till
chin – tin
chip – tip

Chad – tad
chap – tap

chalk – talk
chop – top

chub – tub
chug – tug
Chuck – tuck

chose – toes

chew – two

chide – tide
chime – time

cheer – tier

chair – tear

char – tar
chart – tart

chore – tore

tʃ__ t__ Phrases

choose Todd
cheap talk

cheap tire
chipped tooth

chase toads
China town

Words of Increasing Length and Phrases That Begin with /tʃ/

cheer	cheerful	cheerfully
chair	chairman	chairmanship
child	childish	childishness
challenge	challenger	challengers
chop	choppy	choppy water
chill	chilly	chilly weather
chew	chewing	chewing gum
chick	chicken	chicken feed
chip	chipped	chipped beef
chat	chatter	chatter box
chunk	chunky	chunky chocolate
chart	charter	charter member
check	checker	checker board game
champ	champion	championship match

Sentences with /tʃ/

1. Gotcha!
2. Go inch by inch.
3. Scratch that itch.
4. Jack is such a cheater.
5. He's a charming chap.
6. George cheats at checkers.
7. It's not just chilly, it's frigid!
8. Choose peach pie or chocolate cake.
9. Don't choke on those fish and chips.
10. Too much rich food makes me belch.
11. It's just too chilly at the beach in March.
12. She can choose Dutch apple or peach pie.
13. They shared a huge batch of French fries.
14. Jack cheats at chess every chance he gets.
15. Richard made his fortune as a llama rancher.
16. The coach watched the touchdown and cheered.
17. A bunch of cockroaches just ran under the couch.
18. Jay's matching couch and chair were very cheap.
19. I ate too much of that chocolate chip cookie dough.
20. We chowed down on chicken, pizza, and peach dessert.
21. I just can't watch him put ketchup on his poached eggs.
22. Usually he's at the beach house lounging on the porch, watching the fishing boats.

d__

Dee, deed, deal, dean, deep
ditch, did, dig, Dick, dill, dim, dish
day, Dale, date, Dave, days
Deb, dead, deaf, deck, den, death
dad, dam, Dan, dash
Dutch, dud, dug, duck, dull, dumb, done, dove, does
dog, dodge, dock, doll, dawn, dot
do, dude, duke, duel, doom, dune, deuce, dues
die, died, dial, dime, dine, dice, dive, dyes
dirt
deer
dare
dark, darn, dart
door, dorm

d__ d__ Phrases

dark day
dig deep
dead duck
deep dish
duck down
deep ditch
dive down
Dear Dad
dull day
dog days
D-Day
Dave did
deep down
Dan's den
dip down
dorm door
dooms day
Daffy Duck

__d

bead, deed, feed, heed, lead, need, read, seed, weed

bid, did, hid, kid, lid, rid, Sid

aid, fade, jade, laid, made, paid, raid, shade, wade

Ed, bed, dead, fed, head, led, Ned, red, said, shed, Ted, wed

add, bad, Chad, fad, had, lad, mad, pad, sad

bud, dud, mud

odd, cod, nod, pod, rod, sod, Todd, wad

ode, code, load, mode, road, sewed, showed, toad

good, hood, could, should, would

booed, chewed, dude, food, mood, nude, rude, sued

bowed, loud, vowed

died, guide, hide, lied, ride, side, tide, wide

bird, heard, word

beard, cheered, feared, sheared, weird

dared, cared, shared

guard, hard, card, lard, yard

board, Ford, gourd, cord, lord, poured, roared, sword, ward

__d __d Phrases

Ted lied

sad lad

loud Ford

weird dude

bad feud

odd food

bad seed

food fad

good kid

made bread

Chad cried

red sled

good mood

hard bed

bad blood

need bread

fried food

slurred word

bread board

sled ride

Ned snored

d__ __d Phrases

deep mud

dig sod

dill seed

dog food

death bed

duck food

Doug sued

doubt Ted

deer herd

dull blade

dark red

date bread

d – b Contrasts

Dee - bee
deed - bead
dean - bean
deep - beep

did - bid
dig - big
Dick - Bic
dill - Bill

day - bay
Dale - bale
date - bait
days - bays

dead - bed
den - Ben
death - Beth

dad - bad
dam - bam
Dan - ban
dash - bash

dud - bud
dug - bug
duck - buck
dumb - bum
done - bun
does - buzz

dog - bog
doll - ball
dot - bought

dough - bow

due - boo
dude - booed
doom - boom

doubt - bout

die - buy
dyes - buys

dirt - Bert

deer - beer

dare - bear

dark - bark
darn - barn
dart - Bart

door - bore

d__ b__ Phrases

dull book
Dutch boy
dead beat
dough boy
dead birch
dodge ball

dull boss
deep bay
dog bite
deep bowl
dog bone
dead bear

darn bug
dirt bike
drive by
dart board
dune buggy
Dick's brain

d – g Contrasts

dig - gig
dill - gill

day - gay
Dale - Gayle
dame - game
Dane - gain
date - gate
Dave - gave
daze - gaze

debt - get

dab - gab
dad - gad
dash - gash

dull - gull
dumb - gum
done - gun

dock - gawk
doll - gall
dawn - gone
dot - got

dough - go
Dole - goal
doze - goes

due - goo
duel - ghoul
dune - goon
dupe - goop
deuce - goose

down - gown
doubt - gout

die - guy
died - guide

deer - gear

door - gore

d__ g__ Phrases

deep gash
dead goose
deep gouge
Dan's gone
dial gauge
Dean's gear

d – n Contrasts

Dee - knee
deed - need
deal - kneel

Dick - Nick

Dale - nail
dame - name

dead - Ned
deck - neck
Dell - Nell

Dan - Nan
dash - Nash

dumb - numb
done - none

dock - knock
dot - not

dough - no
doze - nose

do - new
dude - nude
dune - noon
deuce - noose
dues - news

down - noun

dial - Nile
dine - nine
dice - nice

dear - near

d__ n__ Phrases

do not
dull night
done now
did not
dark night
door nail
dare not
dead gnat
does not

d – t Contrasts

Dee – tea
deal - teal
dean – teen

Dick –tick
dill – till
dim – Tim
dip – tip

Dale – tale
dame – tame

dead – Ted
Dell – tell
den – ten

dab – tab
dad – tad
Dan – tan

dub – tub
Dutch – touch
dug – tug
duck – tuck
done – ton

dock – talk
doll – tall
dot – taught

dough – toe
Dole – toll

due – two
duel – tool
doom – tomb
dune – tune

dowel – towel
down – town

die – tie
died – tied
dime – time
dine – tine
dyes – ties

deer – tear

dart – tart

dare – tear

door – tore

d__ t__ Phrases

dart team
dark tan
deep tub
dark tomb
dull tip
dial tone
dead toad
dull tack
Dutch team
duck tail
dull tone
dog tag
dove tail
dark tile
dead tired

dr__

dream
drip
Drake, drain, drape
dread, dress
drab, drag, drat
drug, drudge, drum
drop
drone, drove
drew, drool, droop
dry, dried, drive, dries

Words of Increasing Length and Phrases That Begin with /d/

dirt	dirty	dirtiest
depend	dependable	dependability
develop	development	developmental
danger	dangerous	dangerously
discipline	disciplinary	disciplinarian
demand	demanding	demanding job
discuss	discussion	discussion group
desire	desirable	desirable situation
democrat	democratic	democratic party

Sentences with /d/

1. I do.
2. I did it.
3. I did not.
4. Don't do it.
5. Who did that?
6. I paid my dues.
7. He had it made.
8. Dinner is ready.
9. Don't fall down.
10. He lied; I did not.
11. It's a hot, dry day.
12. Open the door, Ted.
13. I did not do it. She did.
14. Dig the ditch knee deep.
15. Don't dilly-dally around.
16. Hide the beads in the sand.
17. Your date bread is delicious.
18. Don't deal that deck of cards.
19. Feed the ducks from the dock.
20. Don't wade in the mud puddle.
21. He saved every dime he earned.
22. Their double date was a disaster.
23. Did she find the kind she needed?
24. They deliver doughnuts every day.
25. Fried foods are bad for my middle.
26. The chip dip in this dish is delicious.
27. She dyed her hair an odd shade of red.
28. Don't feed Fido that food. It's not fit for a dog.
29. She made the bed, fed the cat, and headed out the door.

f__

fee, feed, feel, feet
fib, fig, fill, fin, fish, fit, fizz
Faye, fade, fake, face, fate, faith, phase
fetch, fell
fad, fan, fat
fudge, fun, fuss, fuzz
fog, fall, fawn, fought
foe, folk, foal, foam, phone
food, fool
full
fuel
foul
file, fine, fight
foil
fur, firm, fern
fear, feared, fierce
fair
far, farm, farce
four, Ford, fork, form, force, fort, fourth

f__ f__ Phrases

fish food
feel fine
four feet
fierce fight
fine food
feel fit
fish face

fat feet
fish farm
full face
fine fudge
feared foe
fine form
foul feet

force feed
fake fur
fish fork
fig farm
fake fight
fine farce
fast food

__f __f Phrases

half off
rough life
tough turf
goof off

half deaf
rough surf
half laugh
tough beef

staff chief
brief life
gruff chef
tough stuff

f__ __f Phrases

fall off
feel safe
fat calf
fine life
far off
fig leaf
fine beef

farm life
fail safe
fade off
full life
fine wife
fight off
fat chef

fourth wife
fine chef
face off
fine staff
feel rough
fake cough
funny stuff

f – p Contrasts

fee - pea
feel - peel
feet - Pete
fees - peas

fig - pig
fill - pill
fin - pin
fit - pit
fix - picks

Faye - pay
fade - paid
fail - pail
feign - pain
face - pace
phase - pays

fad - pad
fan - pan
fang - pang
fat - pat

fun - pun

fall - Paul
fawn - pawn
fought - pot

foal - pole

fool - pool

full - pull

foot - put

few - pew
fuse - pews

foul - Powell

firm - perm

fear - peer
fierce - pierce
fears - peers

fair - pair
fares - pears

far - par

four - pour
Ford - poured
fork - pork
fort - port

f_ p_ Phrases

fine peas	fine putt	four pets
fudge pie	five pies	fake pearl
fine peach	fat pig	fish pond

f – s Contrasts

fee – see
feed – seed
feel – seal
feet – seat
fees – seize

fill – sill
fin – sin
fit – sit

Faye – say
fake – sake

fed – said
fell – sell

fad – sad
fat – sat

fun – sun

fought – sought

foe – sew
phone – sewn

foot – soot

fine – sign
fight – sight

foil – soil

fur – sir

fear – sear

Ford – sword
force – source
fort – sort

f_ s_ Phrases

feel sick	fine suit	fair sky
fine soap	fake sword	four suits
full sail	fire side	five sides
fight song	feel sad	Faye's sad

f_ θ_ Phrases

feel thin	fierce thing	phase three

f – ð Contrasts

fee – thee
fees – these

Faye – they
fade – they'd
fail – they'll

fan – than
fat – that

foe – though
foes – those

fair – their

f__ ð__ Phrases

face them
feed them
feed these
fear them
fear those
phone them

force that
force them
force these
force those
find them
find these

find that
find those
fix them
fix that
fix these
fix those

f – v Contrasts

fee – V
feel – veal

fail – veil
feign – vein
face – vase

fan – van
fat – vat

fawn – Vaughn

foul – vowel

file – vile
fine – vine

fern – Vern

fear – veer
feared – veered

f__ v__ Phrases

fine vase
fat veal
fine verse

fear Val
fourth vote
fight Vern

first vote
first verse
five vases

fl__

flea, fleece, fleas	flub, flood, flush	fly, flight, flies
flick, flip	flock, flop, floss	flare, flares
flame	flow, flowed, float	floor, floors
fleck, fled, flesh	flew, flute	
flab, flag, flap, flash, flat	flower	

fr__

free, freed, freak, freeze	Fred, fresh, fret	fruit
fridge, frill, frizz	Fran, frat	frown
frail, frame, phrase	frog, frock, froth	fry, fried, fright, fries

Words of Increasing Length That Begin with /f/

fun	funny	funnier
fuzz	fuzzy	fuzzier
fish	fishing	fishing pole
fail	failure	failures
fear	fearless	fearlessly
faith	faithful	faithfully
force	forceful	forcefulness
photo	photograph	photographic
fortune	fortunate	fortunately
favor	favorable	favorably
feeble	feebleminded	feeblemindedness

Sentences with /f/

1. Fill it half full.
2. Fee, fie, foe, fum.
3. I fell flat on my duff.
4. I'm feeling fit as a fiddle.
5. I found a four-leaf clover.
6. They flew in from Florida.
7. She's fifty-four, not fifty-five.
8. The fight was fast and furious.
9. I'm very full after all that food.
10. They will float the river on a raft.
11. They have a fish fry every Friday.
12. It's half full, Victor, not half empty.
13. After that fiasco, I feel very foolish.
14. The office staff took the afternoon off.
15. The furnace failed and we nearly froze.
16. All fees were final and due on the fourth.
17. Forget it! Leave! Take off! See if I care!
18. If Patty fails the math final, she's finished!
19. My feet are so fat, they don't fit into my favorite loafers.

g__

geese

gill, give

gay, gauge, Gayle, game, gain, gate, gave, gaze

guess, get

gab, gal, gang, gap, gas, gash

gull, gum, gun, Gus, gush, gut

gob, gawk, gone, gong, got, gauze

go, goal, goat, goes

good

goof, goose

gouge, gown, gout

guy, guide, guys

girl

gear

guard

gore, gourd

g__ g__ Phrases

good game
get gas
good guess
gas gauge
good guide
get gum
good guy
Good grief!
Great guns!

__g

big, dig, fig, pig, rig, wig
egg, beg, keg, leg, Meg, peg
bag, gag, hag, jag, lag, nag, rag, sag, tag, wag
bug, chug, dug, hug, jug, mug, rug, tug, thug
bog, dog, fog, hog, jog, cog, log

__g __g Phrases

big pig
shag rug
big bug
dog tag
big wig
egg nog
big dog
rag bag
big mug
peg leg
big bag
big rig
big hog
big league
big egg

g__ __g Phrases

gas hog
good dog
goose egg

good egg
go dig
guard dog

go jog
go beg
get Doug

g – b Contrasts

gill – bill

gay – bay
Gabe – babe
Gayle – bail
gate – bait
gaze – bays

gas – bass
gash - bash

guess – Bess
get – bet

gum – bum
gun - bun
Gus – bus
gut – but

gob – Bob
got – bought

go – bow
goal – bowl
goat – boat
goes – bows

gout – bout

guy – buy

gear – beer
geared – beard

gore – bore
gourd – bored

g__ b__ Phrases

get back
good book

gone back
good boy

give back
goes by

g – d Contrasts

gill – dill

Gayle – Dale
game – dame
gain – Dane
gait – date
gave – Dave
gaze – daze

get – debt

gab – dab
gash – dash

gull – dull
gum – dumb
gun – done

gall – doll
gone – dawn
got – dot

go – dough
goat – dote
goes – doze

goo – due
goon – dune
goose – deuce

gown – down
gout – doubt

guy – die
guide – died

gear – deer

gore – door

g__ d__ Phrases

good deal
guard dog
good deed
gas deal
get dad
good dog
get done
goose down
good day
guide dog
Go Dave!
Great Dane

g – dʒ Contrasts

gig - jig
gill - Jill
Gayle - jail
gain - Jane
guess - Jess
get - jet
gab - jab
gut - jut
gob - job
gone - John
got - jot
gauze - jaws
go - Joe
goal - Joel
goose - juice
gear - jeer

g__ dʒ__ Phrases

get Jane
good joke
good juice
get Jess
good jazz
gooey jam
great joy
glass jar
Get Jack!

g – k Contrasts

gill - kill
game - came
gain - cane
gave - cave
gab - cab
gal - Cal
gap - cap
gas - Cass
gum - come
gut - cut
gob - cob
gall - call
gone - con
got - cot
gauze - cause
goal - coal
goat - coat
good - could
goo - coo
ghoul - cool
goop - coop
girl - curl
gourd - cord
guard - card

g__ k__ Phrases

gas cap
give cash
good king
gas can
good cause
goose call
good coat
go cart
good cook
gun case
good car
gold coin
golf course
grow corn
great cook
ground corn
golf cart

__g – __ŋ Contrasts

big – Bing
dig – ding
rig – ring
wig – wing
bag – bang
gag – gang
hag – hang
rag – rang
sag – sang
tag – tang
lug – lung
rug – rung
tug – tongue
log – long

__g __ŋ Phrases

big bang
big ring
big fling

gl__

glee, gleam
glib, glitch
glaze
glad, glass
Glenn
glum, glut, glove
glob, gloss
glow, globe, gloat
glue, glued
glide

gr__

greed, grief, Greek, green, grease, greet
grid, grill, grim, grin, grip, grit
gray, grade, grain, grace, grate, grave, graze
grab, grass
grub
grow, groan, gross, growth, grove, grows
grew, groom, groove
grime, gripe

Words of Increasing Length and Phrases That Begin with /g/

govern	government	governmental
grace	graceful	gracefully
grand	granddad	granddaddy
gob	gobbled	gobbledegook
get	get up	get up and go
good	goody	goody-goody
guess	guessing	guessing game
gold	golden	golden gate
gift	gift wrap	gift wrapping

Sentences with /g/

1. Go get gas.
2. Great guns!
3. Kill that ugly bug!
4. Get the tacos to-go.
5. This eggnog is great!
6. Let's go golfing again.
7. Give grandpa a big hug.
8. As snug as a bug in a rug.
9. Come back again in August.
10. Good grief, that game was long!
11. A pink dogwood grows by the gate.
12. Can you grow eggplant in your garden?
13. The hungry pigs gobbled down the corn.
14. Don't forget to get a box of graham crackers.
15. The gardener got that pesky ground hog for good.

h__

he, heel, heap, heat, heave, he's
hitch, hid, hick, hill, him, hip, hit, his
hay, hail, hate, haze
head, heck, hell, hen
hatch, had, half, hack, ham, hash, hat, has
hub, hutch, huff, hug, hull, hum, hush, hut
ha, hog, hall, hop, hot
hood, hoof, hook
who, who'd, who'll, whom, hoop, hoot, whose
Hugh, huge, Hughes
hoe, hole, home, hope, hose
how, howl, house
high, hide, hike, height, hive
her, Herb, heard, hearse, hurt, hers
here
hair
hard, hark, harm, harp, harsh, heart
hoard, horn, horse

h__ h__ Phrases

ha-ha	his heel	he has
he had	hide him	hard head
he hid	his head	huge hole
high horse	haul hay	hot hearth
hothead	ham hock	he's hurt
high hat	hit hard	huge hog
hide him	he's home	her hope
high hill	hard heart	whole heart
he heard	ham hash	huge hat
hard hat	his house	hip-hop
ho-hum	hurt him	hit him
whole hog	hot house	heavy haze

h – j Contrasts

hail - Yale	hack - yak	who'll - you'll
hell - yell	ham - yam	hard - yard
hen - yen	hum - yum	hear - year

h__ j__ Phrases

he yawned	his yacht	Hey! You!
his youth	he's young	hard year
half year	hard yolk	how young

Words of Increasing Length and Phrases That Begin with /h/

hot	hothead	hotheaded
hope	hopeless	hopelessly
hard	harden	hardening
hold	holding	holdings
hand	handcuff	handcuffed
help	helpless	helplessness
health	healthy	healthiest
humid	humidify	humidifier
hard	hardy	hardier
horse	horseman	horsemanship
heed	heedless	heedlessly
hum	humming	humming bird
honey	honeydew	honeydew melon

Sentences with /h/

1. He has it.
2. Ho, ho, ho!
3. Is he home?
4. My head hurts.
5. He's a hothead.
6. She held my hand.
7. I have high hopes.
8. Her house is half his.
9. Hold your head high.
10. Who has a headache?
11. Who hid my Hula-Hoop?
12. She hit him on the head.
13. It hurts to hold my head up.
14. They have a herd of horses.
15. I'll have Harry's hide for this.
16. In her haste, she cut her hand.
17. Hardly any hail hit my house.
18. That ham dinner was ho-hum.
19. How long has she been home?
20. In her heyday, she was a handful.
21. A hush fell over the whole house.
22. She hid in the hen house hoping you would find her.

dʒ__

Jean, jeep, jeans
jig, Jill, gym, gin
Jay, jade, Jake, jail, Jane
Jed, Jeff, gem, Jess, jet
jab, Jack, jam, Jan, jazz
jug
jaw, job, jog, John, jot, jaws
Joe, joke, Joel, Joan, Joe's
jewel, June, juice
joy, join
jerk, germ
jeer
jar

dʒ__ dʒ__ Phrases

jam jar
Joe's Jeep
gin jug
join Jake
Joe's Gym
juice jug
join Gene
join Jack
Jack's Jeep

__dʒ

siege
ridge
age, gauge, cage, page, rage, sage, wage
edge, hedge, ledge, wedge
badge
budge, fudge, nudge
dodge, lodge
huge
gouge
urge, merge, purge, verge
barge, charge, large
forge, gorge

__dʒ __dʒ Phrases

huge ridge
large gouge
huge barge
large bridge
large barge
huge bridge

dʒ__ __dʒ Phrases

jet age
jet gauge
jazz age
Jack's age
Joe's lodge
Jean's Dodge

dʒ – g Contrasts

jig – gig
Jill – gill
Jane – gain
Jess – guess
jet – get
jab – gab
jut – gut
job – gob
John – gone
jot – got
jaws – gauze
Joe – go
Joel – goal
juice – goose
jeer – gear

dʒ – ʃ Contrasts

Jean – sheen
Jeep – sheep
gin – shin
jade – shade
Jake – shake
jail – shale
Jane – Shane
Jed – shed
Jeff – chef
Jack – shack
jam – sham
John – Shawn
Joe – show
Joan – shown
jerk – shirk
jeer – sheer
jar – Char

dʒ__ ʃ__ Phrases

Joe's shoes
Jay's shirt
Joe's shy
Joe's shirt
Jack's shack
Joe's short
Jay's shack
Jeff's short
Jack's shoes

dʒ – tʃ Contrasts

Jeep – cheap
Jill – chill
gin – chin
Jane – chain
Jess – chess
jug – chug
joke – choke

dʒ__ tʃ__ Phrases

Joe's check	Gene's check	Jay's check
Gene cheats	Jay cheats	Joe cheats
Jay's cheap	Joe's cheap	Gene's cheap

dʒ – z Contrasts

gee - Z	Jack - Zach	jar - czar
Jen - Zen	Joan - zone	

Words of Increasing Length and Phrases That Begin with /dʒ/

jab	jabber	jabbering
jay	jaywalk	jaywalker
jug	juggle	juggler
judge	judgment	judgmental
just	justify	justifiable
general	generalize	generalization
jump	jumping	jumping jack
jig	jigsaw	jigsaw puzzle
ginger	gingerbread	gingerbread house
John	Johnny	Johnny Appleseed

Sentences with /dʒ/

1. Jenny's a gem!
2. This job is a joke!
3. I sure enjoy my job.
4. Jack is such a joker.
5. Chill some orange juice.
6. Jot down your job duties.
7. She gave Jack a sharp jab.
8. Jack and Jill jogged up the hill.
9. Put the jelly in these special jars.
10. Angie's happy that Jerry's in jail.
11. That corporation merger is a joke.
12. She jogged over to Gene's house.
13. The giant barge carried a large load.
14. Can you join me at the gym, Chuck?
15. The jet crashed just south of Jackson.
16. His job was to paint the bridge orange.
17. Joe's fish was just a smidgen larger than Jeff's.
18. The shelves were jammed with jars of peach jelly.
19. My old Dodge was crushed by a huge contraption at the junk yard.

k__

key, keen, keep, Keith, keys
kid, kick, kill, Kim, king, kiss, kit
Kay, cage, cake, kale, came, cane, cape, case, Kate, cave
keg, Ken
cab, catch, calf, Cal, can, cap, cash, cat
cub, cuff, come, cup, cut
cob, cod, cough, call, con, cot, cause
code, Coke, coal, comb, cone, coat, cove
coo, cool, coop
could, cook
cube, cute
cow, couch, cows
kite
coy, coil, coin
curb, Kirk, curl, curse, Curt, curve
care, cared, carol, cares
car, card, Carl, carp, cart, carve, cars
core, cord, cork, corn, course, court

k__ k__ Phrases

car coat
key case
can-can
car key
keep cool
cat cage
kite kit
corn cob
call Kim
court cook
cut corn
coal car
Cape Cod
court case
Kate can
coin case
cool cave
card key
cool cat
King Kong
corn curl
cow cart
keep cows
catch cold
cute kid
cut cards
cold cash

__k __k Phrases

teak deck
work week
check back
oak deck
knick-knack
weak back
tick-tock
back pack
bike lock
thick book
look like
cake walk
look back
duck walk
dark lake
bike rack
book work
walk back
knock-knock
book nook
weak neck
take back
bike wreck
fake check
look sick
check mark
talk back
joke book
kick back
chalk mark
sick joke
weak dike
black lake
pork steak
quick hike
bike track
slick rock
take stock
black rock
book clerk
weak brick
sneak peek

k__ __k Phrases

key rack
case book
call back
cool lake
cut back
could talk
car wreck
came back
could leak
cool walk
come look
cup rack
can walk
come back
code book
cake walk
can cook
coat rack
can work
card deck
cup cake
kick back
cake bake
corn stock

k – tʃ Contrasts

keep – cheap
keys – cheese

kick – chick
kill – chill
kin – chin

cane – chain
case – chase

cap – chap
cat – chat

cub – chub
come – chum

Coke – choke

coo – chew

cow – chow

care – chair
cares – chairs

car – char
card – charred

cart – chart

core – chore

k__ tʃ__ Phrases

keep chilled
cute chick

call Chuck
car chase

corn chowder
cook chicken

k – g Contrasts

kill – gill

kale – Gayle
came – game
cane – gain
cape – gape
Kate – gate
cave – gave

cab – gab
Cal – gal
calf – gaff
cap – gap
Cass – gas

come – gum
cuss – Gus
cut – gut

cob – gob
cod – god
call – gall
con – gone
cot – got
cause – gauze

coal – goal
coat – goat

coo – goo
cool – ghoul
coop – goop

curl – girl

card – guard

core – gore
cord – gourd

k__ g__ Phrases

can go
keep guard
card game
cute girl
coast guard
can't go

k – t Contrasts

key – tea
keen – teen
keys – tease

kick – tick
kill – till
Kim – Tim
kin – tin
Kip – tip

cake – take
kale – tail
came – tame
cape – tape

Ken – ten

cab – tab
can – tan
cap – tap

cub – tub

cod – Todd
call – tall
cop – top
cot – taught

cook – took

code – toad
coal – toll
cone – tone
coat – tote

coo – two
cool – tool

kite – tight

coy – toy
coil – toil

care – tear

car – tar
carp – tarp
cart – tart

core – tore
corn – torn
court – torte

k__ t__ Phrases

keep time
can talk
keg tap
could talk
cut teeth
cut tape
kill time
keep ties
come to
cut ties
cold toes
car tools
calm tide
cold tea
keep talking

kl__

clean, cleat
click, clip
clay, claim
clad, clam, clan, clap, class
club, clutch, cluck

claw, clod, clog, clock, cloth, clause
clue, clues
cloak, clone, clothe, clove, close
cloud, clown, clout

clerk
Clyde, climb
clear, cleared
Clare
Clark

kr__

creek, cream, creep, crease
crib, Chris
crane, crate, crave, craze
crab, crack, cram, crash

crutch, crud, crumb, crush
crock, crawl, crop, cross
crow, croak, chrome
crew, crude, cruel, cruise

crouch, crowd, crown
cry, cried, crime, cries

Words of Increasing Length and Phrases That Begin with /k/

car	carsick	carsickness
care	careless	carelessness
captive	captivate	captivating
carbon	carbonate	carbonation
correct	correction	correctional
create	creative	creativity
call	calling	calling card
king	kingdom	kingdom come
cape	Cape Cod	Cape Cod Bay
camp	campfire	Campfire Girls
key	keynote	keynote speaker

Sentences with /k/

1. I like cod.
2. Keep cool, hothead.
3. Can you milk a cow?
4. I can't get a cold now.
5. Take Kevin to the lake.
6. Who likes candy canes?
7. Check back in one week.
8. Can you cook it in a kettle?
9. I like to take walks by the lake.
10. Come back here and take a look.
11. Keep the keys in your coat pocket.
12. The cops took the carjacker to court.
13. She caught a cold and coughed all night.
14. My cubicle at work is cozy, not cramped.
15. Take a break and get some cake and coffee.
16. His kite keeps getting caught in the oak tree.
17. Jack, keep your cash in a bank, not in a shoe box!
18. Check the cookbook before you bake those cookies.
19. Check the back of the box before you bake that chocolate cake.

l__

Lee, leech, lead, leaf, league, leak, lean, leap, lease, leash, leave
lid, lick, limb, Lynn, lip, lit, live, Liz
laid, lake, lame, lane, lace, late
led, leg, ledge, Len, less, let
lab, latch, lad, laugh, lag, lack, lamb, lap, lass
lug, luck, lull, lung, lush, love
lob, log, lodge, lock, lawn, long, lop, loss, lot, laws
low, load, loaf, loan, loathe
lube, lewd, Luke, loon, loop, loose, loot, lose
look
loud, louse, lout
lie, lied, life, like, Lyle, lime, line, lice, light, live
Lloyd, loyal
lurch, learn
leer
lair
lard, large, lark
lore, lord

l__ l__ Phrases

long life
loose lip
loud laugh
light load
lush life
let loose
large lot
long laugh
live long
loose line
life-like
lame leg
long look
low light
life line
large lawn
lay low
leave late
long line
love life
less lard
live life
long leash
less loot
loose latch
live leech
lake lodge
latch lock
lewd look
long ledge
loose lid
less lawn
long lease
large loaf
log lodge
long leap
lame lamb
load logs
long legs
lax line
laugh loudly
live and let live

__l

eel, deal, feel, heel, meal, kneel, peel, real, seal, teal, veal, wheel, zeal

ill, bill, chill, dill, fill, gill, hill, Jill, kill, mill, pill, sill, will

ale, bail, Dale, fail, Gayle, hail, jail, kale, mail, nail, pail, rail, sail, shale, tail, whale, Yale

bell, fell, hell, gel, Nell, sell, shell, tell, well, yell

pal, shall

dull, gull, hull, lull

all, ball, doll, fall, hall, call, mall, Paul, shawl, tall, wall

bowl, Dole, foal, goal, hole, coal, mole, pole, roll, soul, toll

duel, fool, cool, pool, rule, tool

bull, full, pull, wool

owl, bowel, foul, howl, jowl, towel, vowel

dial, file, Lyle, mile, Nile, pile, tile, while

oil, boil, foil, coil, loyal, royal, soil, toil

Earl, girl, curl, pearl, whirl

barrel, carol, peril

Carl

__l __l Phrases

full meal
oil well
mail call
pool hall
heal well
full sail
foul ball
ill will
roll call
whale oil
jail cell
real wool
feel full
wool shawl
feel ill
oil bill
hail fell
boil oil
toll call
tall tale
mole hill
meal hall
Bill fell
tell Neil
real deal
feel well
jail bail
Earl fell
real tall
tall girl
dull file
foul smell
steel wool
small meal
snail shell
steel ball
stale ale
feel small
small wheel
steal mail
stale roll
still full

l__ __l Phrases

loud bell
log pile
long haul
large meal
loose wheel
long nail
lack fuel
log wall
large pearl
long fall
leave jail
late meal

light wool
large pool
look well
lewd call
less coal
large hole
leak oil
long tail
lose mail
large pail
loophole
large bowl

long meal
live well
loud call
large shell
low wall
life goal
large bell
lace shawl
large bill
lone gull
lewd tale
last call

l – n Contrasts

Lee – knee
lead – need
lease – niece

lick – Nick
lip – nip
lit – knit

led – Ned
let – net

lab – nab
lag – nag
lack – knack
lap – nap

lock – knock
lot – not

look – nook

low – know
load – node
loan – known

Lou – new
lewd – nude
loon – noon
loose – noose
loot – newt
lose – news

life – knife
Lyle – Nile
line – nine
lice – nice
light – night

leer – near

l__ n__ Phrases

long night
lame knee
look new
loud knock
long note
loose knit
long nap
look now
less noise

learn now
long neck
look nice
loose noose
laugh now
late night
look neat
long nail
long knife

lug nut
loud noise
long noose
late news
Loch Ness
long nose
love nest
last night
least known

l – r Contrasts

leech – reach
lead – read
leaf – reef
leap – reap

lid – rid
limb – rim
lip – rip

lay – ray
lake – rake
lane – rain
lace – race
late – rate

led – red
Len – wren

lag – rag
lack – rack
lamb – ram
lap – wrap
lash – rash

lug – rug
lush – rush

law – raw
lob – rob
lock – rock
lawn – Ron
loss – Ross
lot – rot

low – row
load – road
loam – roam

lewd – rude
loom – room
loot – root

lie – rye
lied – ride
lime – rhyme
line – Rhine
light – right

leer – rear

lair – rare

lore – roar
lord – roared

l__ r__ Phrases

long run
loose rock
less rain
long robe
large rock
loud ring
long route
lake road
leg race

light ray
long road
long reach
lawn rake
loud roar
left rear
long ride
look right
loose rail

large rose
loose robe
long rice
loud rain
long room
log roll
long rug
large rug
Lee's rude

l__ w__ Contrasts

Lee - we
lead - weed
leak - week
lean - wean
leap - weep
leave - weave

lick - wick
Lynn - win
lit - wit

lay - way
laid - wade
lake - wake
lane - Wayne
late - wait

ledge - wedge
Len - when
let - wet

lock - walk

lie - why
lied - wide
life - wife
line - wine
light - white
lies - wise

lore - war
lord - ward

lair - wear

l__ w__ Phrases

long wait
lead weight
loud whine
long week
loose weave
lack work
live whale

learn why
lawn work
low wall
live wire
lose weight
lab work
long wall

less wheat
long walk
late one
large wall
late walk
light wind
last will

l – j Contrasts

Len – yen
less – yes
let – yet

lack – yak
lamb – yam

lung – young

lawn – yawn
lot – yacht

learn – yearn

leer – year

lore – your

l__ j__ Phrases

loud yell
large yacht
look young
loud yawn

light-year
lush yard
like you
long yard

lost youth
last year
large yam
loose yarn

Words of Increasing Length and Phrases That Begin with /l/

luck	lucky	luckier
like	likely	likelihood
length	lengthy	lengthiest
legal	legalize	legalization
lecture	lecturer	lecturers
local	localize	localization
left	left-hand	left-handed
light	lightning	lightning rod
laugh	laughing	laughing stock
lunch	luncheon	luncheon menu

Sentences with /l/

1. All's well.
2. Neil will, also.
3. Let the ball roll.
4. Look out below.
5. All hell broke lose.
6. Don't lose your cool.
7. The trail led to a lake.
8. Laura felt very foolish.
9. All's well that ends well.
10. Well, Lilly, what will it be?
11. Nick longed for his lost love.
12. A large log blocked the road.
13. It looks real, but it's only glass.
14. Molly will laugh when I tell her.
15. Light the candle on the round table.
16. If you fall in the lake, you better yell.
17. Will you install a rail around the pool?
18. Little Ned likes to blow bubbles all day.
19. The lake was so still it looked like glass.
20. Sandy, I believe you belong in the left lane.
21. He left his life in the limelight to work in a dull flour mill.
22. If Uncle Rudy learns about the lie, he'll leave you out of the will.

m__

me, meal, mean, meet
Mitch, Mick, mill, miss, mitt, myth, Ms.
may, made, make, mail, maim, main, mayor, mate, maze
men, mess, mesh, met
match, mad, Mac, ma'am, man, map, mass, mash, mat, math
much, mud, muck, muss, mush, mutt
ma, mob, mall, mom, moss, moth
mow, mode, mole, moan, moat
mooch, mood, moon, moose, move
mute
mouse
my, Mike, mile, mime, mine, mice, might
merge
mere
mare
mar, march, Marge, mark, marsh, mart, Marv, Mars

m__ m__

moon men	make more	main match
meet me	moose meat	more math
mad men	mean mob	mere men
my mess	my mail	move mom
mad mob	mock me	meet me
meet mom	more men	mesh mat
man made	my mark	main meal
mass mail	more meat	mean mood
mean man	much more	mad maid
my map	mile march	morning mush

__m

beam, ream, seem, team

dim, him, gym, Kim, limb, rim, Tim, whim

aim, dame, fame, game, came, lame, maim, name, same, shame, tame

hem, gem, them

am, dam, ham, jam, lamb, ram, Sam, yam, wham

bum, chum, dumb, gum, hum, come, mum, numb, rum, some

bomb, mom, Tom

dome, foam, home, comb, loam, roam

boom, doom, loom, room, tomb, womb, zoom

fume

I'm, chime, dime, lime, rhyme, time

firm, germ, term, worm

arm, charm, farm, harm

dorm, form, warm

__m __m Phrases

home team
same name
harm him
time bomb
come home
same time
home room
some time
numb arm
same farm
time them
tame him
dim beam
I'm game
some time
charm them

same game
dim room
came home
same theme
I'm Sam
dorm room
home game
harm them
same room
I'm home
charm him
home gym
shame him
lame lamb
lime gum
worm farm

Tom swam
slim Jim
dream home
dumb scheme
blame him
trim form
groom him
time frame
trim them
prime time
blame mom
blame them
same scheme
blame Tom
frame him
steam them

m__ __m Phrases

meet him	my home	made them
moon beam	more charm	my farm
move them	main team	more harm
made some	mail them	merge them
main room	met him	march home
my farm	may seem	mourn him
meal time	my thumb	my dream
math game	make them	my plum
miss him	mad team	mad scheme
mud dam	match him	my drum
my dime	move some	mile swim
miss them	my charm	my claim
meet Kim	might seem	make steam
match game	make some	my crime
move him	my game	mail scam

m – b Contrasts

me - be
meek - beak
mean - bean
meet - beet

mill - bill
mitt - bit

may - bay
make - bake
mail - bail
mace - base
mate - bait

Meg - beg
Mel - bell
men - been
mess - Bess
met - bet

match - batch
mad - bad
Madge - badge
Mac - back
man - ban
mass - bass
mash - bash
mat - bat

mud - bud
muff - buff
mug - bug
muck - buck
mum - bum
mutt - but

ma - baa
mob - Bob
mall - ball
mom - bomb
mop - bop
moss - boss

mow - bow
mole - bowl
moan - bone
moat - boat

moo - boo
mood - booed
moon - boon
moot - boot

mute - butte

my - by
Mike - bike
might - bite

mere - beer

mare - bear

Marge - barge
mark - bark

more - bore

m__ b__ Phrases

mud bath
mean boy
mail bag
moon beam
march back

my bike
more boys
math book
my boat
match book

mud ball
might be
move back
make beds
my brain

Words of Increasing Length That Begin with /m/

mean	meaning	meaningful
mount	mountain	mountaineer
math	mathematic	mathematical
murder	murderer	murderers
moment	momentary	momentarily
market	marketable	marketability
music	musical	musically
myth	mythologic	mythological
magnet	magnetic	magnetically
mechanic	mechanical	mechanically
maneuver	maneuverable	maneuverability
mystery	mysterious	mysteriously

Sentences with /m/

1. I met my match.
2. My arm is numb.
3. I miss my hometown.
4. I've made up my mind.
5. I'm moving back home.
6. Come with me, my dear.
7. She came home in a bad mood.
8. My home gym is mighty dusty.
9. Make some lemon meringue pies.
10. I make marmalade in the summer.
11. Come to my summer home up north.
12. Our team plays the Mets on Monday.
13. He made a name for himself in B movies.
14. That poor man was no match for the mob.
15. A woman came out screaming bloody murder.
16. I made a mountain of mincemeat and a big mess.
17. Bonnie came home from the mall without a dime.
18. Meet me by my locker at the same time tomorrow.
19. It was Mary who made me run home to my mother.
20. She demanded I remove my stinky shoes from the room.

n__

knee, need, kneel, niece, neat, knees

Nick, nip, knit

nail

Ned, neck, Nell, net

nab, nag, nap, gnat

nudge, numb, none, nut

knob, notch, nod, knock, not

no, known, note, nose

new, nude, noon, noose, newt, news

nook

now, noun

knife, Nile, nine, nice, night

noise

nurse

near

n__ n__ Phrases

knock knees	numb knee	not nice
noon nap	knick-knack	no noise
knock-knock	near noon	new knife
no news	new niece	night nurse
nice night	not known	nag Ned
not new	numb nose	nine notches
no name	new name	nightly news
not now	nice note	No, Nancy!

__n

bean, dean, Jean, keen, lean, mean, seen, sheen, teen, wean

bin, chin, fin, gin, Lynn, pin, sin, shin, tin, thin, win

chain, gain, Jane, cane, lane, main, pain, rain, sane, Shane, vein

Ben, den, hen, Ken, Len, men, pen, wren, ten, then, when

Ann, Dan, fan, can, man, pan, ran, tan, van

bun, done, fun, gun, none, pun, run, sun, shun, ton, one

dawn, fawn, gone, John, con, lawn, pawn, Ron, Shawn, Vaughn

bone, phone, Joan, cone, loan, moan, sewn, shown, tone

boon, dune, June, loon, moon, noon, soon, tune

down, gown, noun, town

dine, fine, line, mine, nine, pine, sign, shine, vine, whine

join, coin, loin

earn, burn, fern, learn, turn

barn, darn, yarn

born, horn, corn, Lorne, mourn, torn, thorn, worn

__n __n Phrases

corn bin
one coin
tin can
moon men
ten pin
gone soon
fine tune
main phone
turn sign
burn down
tin horn
vain man
worn thin
turn down
fine yarn
win one
join in
main line
mean man
shin bone
fine line
pine cone
pin down
one phone
con man
sun shown
torn gown
worn down
teen scene
tin pan
one man
sane man
lone pine
torn down
ten ton
John won
thin man
worn coin
one ton
June moon
Gene ran
one town
tin man
one chain
main man
thin bone
Dan won
can run
fine man
join Joan
thin skin
main train
green bean
wine stain
stern man
green lawn
clean fun
grown men
green fern
spin yarn
tin grin
brain scan
brain drain

n__ __n Phrases

need rain
knock down
new moon
not done
no one
nail down
not seen
no rain
new man
not mine
neck chain
kneel down
not vain

nice town
no sign
near win
not sewn
need yarn
knee bone
nine men
not torn
nice lawn
name one
neck vein
not soon
numb shin

no fun
new gown
not one
no wine
near noon
not fun
new barn
nudge Joan
new phone
not green
new stain
not stern
no whining

n – d Contrasts

knee - Dee
need - deed
Neal - deal

Nick - Dick

nail - Dale

Ned - dead
neck - deck
Nell - Dell

Nan - Dan

numb - dumb
none - done

knock - dock
not - dot

no - dough
nose - doze

new - do
nude - dude
noon - dune
noose - deuce
news - dues

noun - down

nice - dice
Nile - dial
nine - dine

near - dear

n – d Phrases

knee deep
near death
new deal
near dawn

nice day
new dad
nail down
new day

nine days
near dark
new deed
knock down

n – l Contrasts

knee - Lee
need - lead
niece - lease

Nick - lick
nip - lip
knit - lit

Ned - led
net - let

nab - lab
nag - lag
knack - lack
nap - lap

knock - lock
not - lot

know - low
known - loan

new - Lou
noon - loon
noose - loose
news - lose

nook - look

knife - life
Nile - Lyle
nice - lice
night - light

near - leer

n__ l__ Phrases

no luck
neat lawn
need less
no light
new lawn
not loud

no loss
need light
not large
need luck
not loyal
night light

new look
new life
not long
night life
nine lives
never lie

n – t Contrasts

knee – tea
kneel – teal
knees – tease

Nick – tick
nip – tip

nail – tail
name – tame

Ned – Ted
Nell – tell

nab – tab
knack – tack

nub – tub
none – ton

nod – Todd
knock – talk
not – taught

nook – took

no – toe
known – tone
note – tote

nose – toes

new – two
noon – tune

noun – town

Nile – tile
night – tight

noise – toys

near – tear

n__ t__ Phrases

nice time
neat town
need time
neck tie
nag Tom

numb toe
nap time
nine teeth
no time
no tip

nice touch
noon time
nine toes
no tone
new toy

__n – __ŋ Contrasts

bin – Bing
din – ding
kin – king
pin – ping
sin – sing
tin – ting
win – wing

ban – bang
fan – fang
pan – pang
ran – rang
tan – tang

run – rung
sun – sung
ton – tongue

gone – gong
lawn – long
Ron – wrong

__n __ŋ Phrases

learn young	one song	plain song
mean gang	fine king	one fling
phone rang	lawn swing	green string

Words of Increasing Length and Phrases That Begin with /n/

nut	nutty	nuttiest
new	newly	newlywed
need	needy	needier
norm	normal	normally
north	northern	Northerner
nerve	nervous	nervously
noise	noisy	noisiness
news	newspaper	newspaperman
note	noteworthy	noteworthiness
north	northwest	northwestern
nine	nineteen	nineteenth
notice	noticeable	noticeably
navigate	navigation	navigational
nine	ninety	ninety-nine
new	New Year's	New Year's Day
night	night watch	night watchman
never	never-never	never-never land
next	next-door	next-door-neighbor

Sentences with /n/

1. I need a nap.
2. Turn on the fan.
3. It's raining again.
4. Oh, no, not again!
5. Turn it down now.
6. Don't turn around.
7. I cannot find the phone.
8. Now I'm the one in pain.
9. My lawn needs lots of rain.
10. Linda ran for Senate and won.
11. They went on their honeymoon.
12. Tom can tune a piano in no time.
13. I'm a mean, lean, running machine.
14. I painted my new barn in only one day.
15. Not one of them was seen before noon.
16. Do you know the man in the next room?
17. The news was not on channel nine tonight.
18. The chicken noodle soup is nearly all gone.
19. I cannot chin myself like when I was young.
20. My old van is nothing more than a noisy tin can.
21. Take the pan of brownies to the dining room and dig in.

__ŋ

king, Ming, ring, sing, thing, wing, zing
bang, fang, gang, hang, rang, sang
lung, rung, sung, tongue, young
gong, long, wrong, song, tong

__ŋ __ŋ Phrases

ding-dong
Hong Kong
wing-ding
King Kong

wrong ring
long fang
wrong king
ping-pong

wrong song
young king
bang-bang
King Kong's long gone

__ŋ – __g Contrasts

Bing – big
ring – rig
wing – wig

bang – bag
gang – gag
hang – hag
rang – rag
sang – sag
tang – tag

lung – lug
rung – rug
tongue – tug

long – log

__ŋ – __n Contrasts

king – kin
sing – sin
ting – tin
wing – win

bang – ban
fang – fan
pang – pan
rang – ran
tang – tan

rung – run
sung – sun
tongue – ton

gong – gone
long – lawn
wrong – Ron

__ŋ __n Phrases

king pin	long gone	long train
wrong one	young man	bowling pin
hang on	long gown	in a long line
wrong line	bring one	bring a sign along

Sentences with /ŋ/

1. Sing a song.
2. She sang the wrong song.
3. If you can't sing it, wing it.
4. The phone rang for a long time.
5. I play ping-pong like a ding-dong.
6. You've got great lungs for singing!
7. The chain gang sang every morning.
8. In spring the wrens sing all day long.
9. He was on a chain gang at Sing-Sing.
10. Playing ping-pong makes me hungry.
11. If that ding-a-ling calls again, hang up.
12. How long were we walking along the lake?
13. Bring those hungry monkeys something to eat.

p__

pea, peach, peak, peel, peep, peace, Pete, peeve, peas
pitch, pig, pick, pill, pin, pit
pay, paid, pale, pain, pace, pave
peg, pen, pep, pet
patch, pad, pack, pal, Pam, pan, pang, pass, pat, path
pub, puff, pun, pup, pus, putt
paw, pod, Paul, pawn, pop, pot, pause
poach, poke, pole, pope, pose
pooch, pool
pull, push, put
pow, pouch, power
pie, pike, pile, pine, pipe, pies
perch, perk, pearl, purse
peer, pierce, peers
pear, pears
par, parch, park, part
pour, poured, pork, port
poor

p__ p__ Phrases

peach pie
pea pod
pen pal
pain pill
peach pit
pay Pete
pig pen
push pin

ping-pong
pie pan
pet peeve
pick pears
pea patch
pay Paul
push-pull
pet pig

pour pop
Pete paid
pick peas
Pike's Peak
play Pitch
pick peaches
pea picker
potato patch

__p

beep, cheap, deep, heap, Jeep, keep, leap, peep, reap, seep, sheep, weep

chip, dip, hip, lip, nip, rip, sip, ship, tip, whip, zip

ape, gape, cape, shape, tape

peg, pen, pep, pet

chap, gap, cap, lap, map, nap, wrap, sap, tap

up, cup, pup

bop, chop, hop, cop, lop, mop, pop, shop, top

hope, cope, mope, pope, rope, soap

goop, hoop, coop, loop, soup

pipe, ripe, type, wipe

burp, chirp

harp, carp, sharp, tarp

__p __p Phrases

keep up
beep-beep
hip deep
tip-top
zip up
keep shop
wrap up
lap top
sharp tip
ship-shape
hip-hop
sip soup
mop up
tap-tap
leap up
deep gap

rip up
chip dip
pop up
top shape
hop up
shape up
chop-chop
mop top
heap up
hip-hip
pep up
cheap Jeep
sharp chap
whip up
pop top
chirp-chirp

wipe up
creep up
top cop
flip up
cheap trip
deep sleep
slurp up
scoop up
stop gap
snap up
swap shop
sweep up
top step
slip up
steep slope
flip-flop

p__ __p Phrases

pea soup
pick up
peace pipe
put up
pork chop
pin up

pet shop
pack up
pitch pipe
push up
pawn shop
pull up

pile up
paid up
puff up
pea crop
potato chip
potato crop

p – b Contrasts

pea -bee
peach - beach
peak - beak
peep - beep
Pete - beat
peas - bees

pig - big
pill - bill
pin - bin
pit - bit

pale - bale
pays - bays

peg - beg
pen - Ben
pet - bet

patch - batch
pad - bad
pack - back
pan - ban
pass - bass
pat - bat
path - bath

pub - bub
puff - buff
pun - bun
pus - bus
putt - but

Paul - ball
pop - bop
pot - bought

pull - bull

pie - buy
pike - bike

perch - birch

par - bar
park - bark
part - Bart

p__ b__ Phrases

pay back
pet bird
peach bin
pale boy
pull back
pine box

pork bone
put back
puff ball
pay bail
peel back
poor boy

push back
pay bills
park board
pear box
park bench
play ball

p – f Contrasts

pea - fee
peel - feel
Pete - feet
peas - fees

pig - fig
pill - fill
pin - fin
pit - fit

pay - Faye
paid - fade
pail - fail
pace - face
pays - phase

pad - fad
pan - fan
pang - fang
pat - fat

pun - fun
pus - fuss

Paul - fall
pawn - fawn
pot - fought

pool - fool

pull - full

pew - few
pew - fuse

Powell - foul

pile - file
pine - fine

perm - firm

peer - fear

par - far

pour - four
poured - Ford
pork - fork
port - fort

pair - fair
pears - fares

p__ f__ Phrases

poor Faye
pick four
push far

paid fee
pet food
pale face

poor food
pay first
play first

p – t Contrasts

pea - tea
peach - teach
peak - teak
peel - teal
peas - tease

pick - tick
pill - till
pin - tin

pale - tail

peck - tech
pen - ten

pad - tad
pack - tack
pan - tan
pang - tang

pod - Todd

pub - tub
pun - ton

Paul - tall
pop - top
pot - tot

poll - toll
pope - taupe
pose - toes

pool - tool

pie - tie
pile - tile
pipe - type
pies - ties

peer - tier
peers - tears

pair - tear

par - tar
part - tart

pore - tore
porch - torch
port - torte

power - tower

p__ t__ Phrases

peach tart
pull tab
pine tree
pause time

pop tune
pool time
pear tree
pure tone

pour tea
pop tart
peach tree
polo team

pl__

plea, plead, please
plaid, plaque, plan

plum, plush
plod, plot

plane, place, plate

pr__

preach	pro, probe	pry, pride, prime, prize
press	proof, prune	
prod, prom, prawn, prop	pray, praise	

Words of Increasing Length and Phrases That Begin with /p/

pig	piggy	piggyback
pack	package	packaging
push	pushy	pushiness
peace	peaceful	peacefully
pep	pepper	peppercorn
pole	polar	polarize
part	partner	partnership
perk	perky	perkier
power	powerful	powerfully
person	personal	personalize
purpose	purposeful	purposefully
period	periodic	periodical
perfect	perfection	perfectionist
planet	planetary	planetarium
problem	problematic	problematical
prison	prisoner	prisoner of war
print	printing	printing press

Sentences with /p/

1. Pardon my pun.
2. Pony up, partner.
3. Pick a big peach.
4. Shape up or ship out.
5. Pour maple syrup on top.
6. Pick only the ripe apples.
7. A cup of bean soup, please.
8. Mom, please pass the pepper.
9. Push and pull it into position.
10. He paid plenty for that carpet.
11. Put the cups and plates up here.
12. Perhaps she will play the piano.
13. Mmm . . . pork chops for supper.
14. She performed her part perfectly.
15. She put a penny in my piggy bank.
16. The pots and pans are piled in a big heap.
17. Peter Piper picked a peck of pickled peppers.
18. I'm hip deep in bills with no hope of paying them.
19. Put the papers on the table and put my pen on top.
20. Mom, after supper I want the biggest piece of peach pie!

r_

reach, reed, reef, reel, ream, reap, wreath

rib, rich, rid, Rick, rim, ring, rip

ray, raid, rage, rake, rail, rain, rang, race, rate, raise

red, wreck, wren

rag, rack, ram, ran, wrap, rash, rat

rub, rough, rug, rum, run, rung, rush, rut

rob, rod, rock, Ron, wrong, Ross, rot

row, robe, roach, road, rogue, roll, roam, rope, wrote, rose

rude, roof, rule, room, root

rye, ride, ripe, rice, right, rise

Roy

rear

rare

roar

r__ r__ Phrases

red rug
rat race
rear room
rough road
red rash
road race
wrong route
red rose
rough ride
wrong road

real rough
red robe
room rate
rim rock
rare rose
right rear
rare rock
wrong room
red wren
rec room

real rich
roof rack
right rim
real rare
wrong rule
rear row
right road
rob Rick
rule Rome
raise rates

r – l Contrasts

reach - leech
reed - lead
reef - leaf
reek - leak
reap - leap

rid - lid
rim - limb
rip - lip

ray - lay
rake - lake
rain - lane
race - lace
rate - late

red - led
wren - Len

rag - lag
rack - lack
ram - lamb
wrap - lap
rash - lash

rug - lug
rush - lush

rob - lob
rock - lock
Ron - lawn
Ross - loss
rot - lot

row - low
road - load

rude - lewd
room - loom
root - loot

rye - lie
ride - lied
rhyme - lime
Rhine - line
right - light

rear - leer
reared - leered

rare - lair

roar - lore

r__ l__ Phrases

rough life
red leaf
real loud
run late

rock ledge
real life
wrong leg
rich life

right leg
rip loose
right lung
righteous lady

r – w Contrasts

reed - weed
reek - week
reel - wheel
reap - weep

rich - witch
rig - wig
Rick - wick
rim - whim
ring - wing
rip - whip

ray - way
raid - wade
rage - wage
rake - wake
rail - whale
rain - Wayne
rate - wait
raise - ways

red - wed
wren - when

rag - wag
rack - whack
ram - wham

run - one
rut - what

rock - walk

row - woe
rose - woes

room - womb

rye - why
ride - wide
Rhine - wine
ripe - wipe
right - white
rise - wise

rear - we're

rare - wear

roar - war

r__ w__ Phrases

right way
red wine
reach one
Rick will
right one

wrong way
ring worm
red wool
rough week
red wood

rough walk
rare one
road way
wrong one
rough work

r – j Contrasts

rude – you'd

wren – yen
Rhett – yet

rack – yak
ram – yam
rap – yap

rung – young

Ron – yawn
rot – yacht

rude – you'd
rule – you'll
Ruth – youth

rail – Yale

rear – year

roar – your

r__ j__ Phrases

rough year
rich yield

raise yams
wrecked yacht

really young

Words of Increasing Length and Phrases That Begin with /r/

rail	railroad	railroading
real	realize	realization
right	righteous	righteousness
rare	rarity	rarities
real	realist	realistic
react	reaction	reactionary
run	runner	runner-up
red	redhead	red-headed
run	running	running leap
read	reading	reading room
rain	rainbow	rainbow trout
remark	remarkable	remarkably
retain	retaining	retaining wall
rhythm	rhythmic	rhythmical
rattle	rattlebrain	rattlebrained
remark	remarkable	remarkably
reason	reasonable	reasonably
reassure	reassuring	reassuringly
recreate	recreation	recreational
resource	resourceful	resourcefully

Sentences with /r/

The /ɝ/ sound and variations of it are presented in the Vowels and Diphthongs Chapter.

1. Run, Randy, run.
2. It rolled across the room.
3. Row, row, row your boat.
4. Her red dress was rather risqué.
5. He raced the raft down the river.
6. They will raise raisin prices soon.
7. Railroads criss-cross the country.
8. O, my love is like a red, red rose.
9. The kids ran around the rec room.
10. The price of real estate is ridiculous.
11. It was a red cherry Tootsie Roll Pop.
12. Robert was raised in the Red River Valley.
13. Ray's place was ransacked by rowdy robbers.
14. Wild mules roam the rugged range of Arizona.

s__

see, seed, seek, seal, seem, seen, seep, cease, seat, seize

Sid, sick, sill, sin, sip, sis, sit

say, safe, sage, sake, sail, same, sane, save

said, sell, set, says

sad, sag, sack, Sam, sap, sass, sat, salve

sub, such, suck, some, sun, sung

saw, sob, sod, sock, song, sauce

so, sewed, soak, soul, soap, sews

Sue, soon, soup, suit, soothe

sow, sour, south, sows

sigh, side, sign, sight, size

soy, soil

sir, search, surge

sore, sword, sort

s__ s__ Phrases

sad sigh
soul search
sad sight
same song
sight see
sad soul
Sue sews
same side
sad scene
soothe Sid
sad sack
sad sum

soap suds
save souls
suit size
save some
said so
some sun
sad sack
soy sauce
set sail
sell some
sun suit
sad song

sail south
safe side
say so
sell soap
South Sea
sip soup
so-so
soft soap
sing songs
send some
sell suits
slippery slope

__s

geese, lease, niece, peace, cease

hiss, kiss, miss, sis, this

ace, base, chase, face, case, lace, mace, pace, race, vase

Bess, guess, less, mess, Tess

bass, gas, mass, pass, sass

us, bus, fuss, Gus, cuss, muss, pus, Russ

boss, loss, moss, Ross, sauce, toss

deuce, goose, juice, loose, moose, noose

house, louse, mouse

ice, dice, lice, mice, nice, rice, vice

choice, voice

hearse, curse, nurse, terse, verse, worse

fierce, pierce

farce

force, horse, course, Morse, source

__s __s Phrases

nice house
less fuss
bus pass
less mess
miss us
race horse
chess piece
house lease
pass us
horse race
gas lease
fierce boss
choice goose

nice voice
chase geese
nice boss
choice rice
hoarse voice
nice niece
less force
race course
Yes, Boss!
terse verse
glass vase
lease space
lace blouse

miss class
bless us
lace dress
less space
gas price
chase us
press pass
brass vase
base price
space race
less spice
goose grease
race tracks

s__ __s Phrases

sea horse
sell less
sour juice
sad face
same bus
some rice
soy sauce
same case
sell gas
set course
same lease
seek peace
same source

sad voice
sea bass
safe house
set loose
some lace
sour face
save less
same voice
sick horse
some gas
sod house
sell ice
same verse

some mice
save face
sad verse
sick niece
say yes
set price
some grease
sale price
safe place
same price
some space
same source
sunny space

s – f Contrasts

see – fee
seed – feed
seal – feel
seat – feet
seize – fees

sill – fill
sin – fin
sit – fit

say – Faye
sake – fake

said – fed
sell – fell

sad – fad
sat – fat

sun – fun

sew – foe
sewn – phone

soot – foot

sign – fine
sight – fight

soil – foil

sir – fur

sear – fear

sword – Ford
source – force
sort – fort

s__ f__ Phrases

see fit
sick fish
some fog
sad face
sword fight
some fish
soak feet
sun fish
some food
snug fit
search far
stood firm
stand firm
save face
cease fighting

s – ʃ Contrasts

see – she
seen – sheen
seep – sheep
seat – sheet

sin – shin
sip – ship

sake – shake
sail – shale
same – shame
sane – Shane
save – shave

said – shed
sell – shell

sack – shack
Sam – sham

sun – shun

sod – shod
sock – shock
Saul – shawl
sop – shop
sought – shot

sew – show
sewed – showed
sews – shows

sue – shoe
suit – shoot

sour – shower
soured – showered

sigh – shy
sign – shine

sir – sure

sore – shore
sort – short

s__ ʃ__ Phrases

sea shell
some shoes
sea shore
sad show
sore shin
sign shop
sad shape
sick sheep
seed shed
side show
same shoe
save shells
suede shoes
six sharks
saddle shoes

s – t Contrasts

sea - tea
seek - teak
seem - team
seen - teen
seize - tease

sick - tick
sill - till
sin - tin
sip - tip

sake - take
sail - tail
same - tame

said - Ted
sell - tell

sad - tad
sag - tag
sack - tack
sap - tap

sub - tub
such - touch
sun - ton
sung - tongue

sod - Todd
sock - talk
song - tong
sop - top
sauce - toss

so - toe
sewed - towed
soul - toll
sewn - tone
sews - toes

sue - two
soon - tune
suit - toot

sigh - tie
side - tide
sign - tine
sight - tight
size - ties

soy - toy
soil - toil

seer - tear

sore - tore
sort - torte

sour - tower

s__ t__ Phrases

same time
sell tea
sword tip
sob tears
sell ten
sad tune
sell tin
size ten
side talk

sore toe
some tape
sip tea
size two
same tire
sage tea
same team
soup tin
such talk

so tall
sore tongue
sit tall
same toe
sad tale
sell toys
set time
sour tart
some tax

s – θ Contrasts

seem – theme
sick – thick
sin – thin
sing – thing

saw – thaw
sought – thought
song – thong

some – thumb
sigh – thigh

s__ θ__ Phrases

same theme
sad thing
sore thigh

same thing
sad theme
seem thick

sad thought
sell things
sore thumb

__s – __θ Contrasts

miss – myth
Bess – Beth
face – faith

bass – bath
mass – math
pass – path
moss – moth

mouse – mouth
worse – worth
force – fourth

__s __θ Phrases

nice teeth
face south
loose tooth

less math
loose mouth
face north

moose teeth
face south
false teeth

s – z Contrasts

see – Z
seal – zeal

sing – zing
sip – zip

sue – zoo
sewn – zone

s__ z__ Phrases

some zip

such zeal

safe zone

sk__

ski, scheme, skis
skid, skill, skim, skin, skip, skit
scale, skate
scab, scam, scan
scuff, skull, scum

Scotch, scoff, Scott
scone, scope
scoop, scoot
sky
scout

scare, scared
scar, scarred
score, scored

sl__

sleek, sleep, sleet, sleeve
slid, slick, slim, sling, slip, slit
slate
sled, sledge

slab, slack, slam, slang, slap, slash
slug, sludge, slum, slush
slob, slop, slot

slow, slope
sloop
sly, slide, slime, slice, slight
slur, slurp

sm__

smell
smack, smash
smug, smudge
smoke

smog, smock, small
smoke
smooch, smooth
smile

smirk
smart

sn__

sneak, sneeze
sniff, snip
snake, snail
snag, snack, snap

snub, snuff, snug
snob, snot
snow, snows
snoop, snooze

snout
snare
sneer
snore

sp__

speech, speed, speak
spill, spin, spit
spade, Spain, space
sped, speck, spell
Spam, spat
spud, spun

spa, spot
spoke
spoof, spook, spool, spoon
spout
spy, spied, spike, spine, spite, spies

spoil
spur, spurt
spear
spare

st__

steed, steel, steam, steep, Steve
stiff, stick, sting, still
stay, stayed, stage, steak, stale, stain, state, stays
stem, step
stab, staff, stag, stack, Stan

stub, stuff, stuck, stung
stock, stall, stop
stow, stole, stone, stove
stew, stool
stood
stout

sty, style, stein
stir, stirred
steer, steered
stare, stared
star, starch, stark, start
store, storm, stored

sw__

Swede, sweep, sweet
switch, swig, swill, swim, swing, Swiss, swish
sway, swayed

swell, sweat
swam
swum, swung
swab, swan, swap, swat, suave

swoon, swoop
swine, swipe
swerve
swear

str__

streak, stream, street
string, strip
stray, strain, straight
stretch, stress

strap
struck, strum, strung, strut
stroke, stroll
straw, strong

stride, strife, strike, stripe, strive

Words of Increasing Length and Phrases That Begin with /s/

save	saving	savings
soap	soapy	soapiness
sea	seasick	seasickness
serve	service	serviceman
sea	seaworthy	seaworthiness
south	southwest	southwestern
sense	sensible	sensibility
safe	safety	safety pin
sand	sandbox	sandbox toy
season	seasoning	seasoning salt
select	selective	selective service
saber	saber-toothed	saber-toothed tiger
senate	senator	senatorial
sorrow	sorrowful	sorrowfully
surprise	surprising	surprisingly
survive	survivor	survivors

Sentences with /s/

1. Sink or swim.
2. The soup was so-so.
3. She sang two songs.
4. The sale is on Saturday.
5. We saw the city by bus.
6. The lemon soda was so sour.
7. They sat beside her on the sofa.
8. It's a juicy snack, but too sweet!
9. They say it is safe to swim there.
10. That scent was so sweet I got sick.
11. The school kids sang at the contest.
12. Wipe that smug smile off your face!
13. The ship sank off the coast of Spain.
14. She ate so many sweets she got sick.
15. He sold topsoil for five dollars a sack.
16. They sang lots of funny songs after supper.
17. The Super Sale is from five to seven on Sunday.
18. His shaky voice was a sure sign he was nervous.
19. The vase was in a safe location on the second shelf.
20. When Sam made a pass at my niece, she smacked him.

ʃ__

she, sheen, sheep, sheet
shade, shake, shale, shame, Shane, shape, shave
shed, shell
shack, shall
shun, shut, shove
shock, shawl, Shawn, shop, shot
show, showed, shown, shows
shoe, shoot, shoes
should, shook
shout
shy, shine
sure, shirt
sheer, sheered
share, shared
shark, sharp
shore, short, shores

ʃ__ ʃ__ *Phrases*

ship-shape
sure shot
she shook
short sheet
shell shock
short shirt
shear sheep
shoe shine
should shave
short shoe
she should
shoe shop
sheep shed
shine shoes
sheep shears
sheer sheet
shiny shoes
Shawn shouted

__ʃ

dish, fish, wish
mesh
ash, cash, dash, hash, mash, sash
gosh, Josh, wash
hush, lush, mush, rush
bush
harsh

ʃ__ __ʃ Phrases

short leash
shell fish
sheer mesh
shell dish
sure fresh
short on cash

ʃ – s Contrasts

she – see
sheen – seen
sheep – seep
sheet – seat

shin – sin
ship – sip

shake – sake
shale – sale
shame – same
Shane – sane
shave – save

shed – said
shell – sell

shack – sack
sham – Sam

shun – sun

shod – sod
shock – sock
shawl – Saul
shop – sop

show – sew
showed – sewed
shows – sews

shoe – sue
shoot – suit

shower – sour

shy – sigh
shine – sign

sure – sir

shore – sore

ʃ__ s__ Phrases

shoe size
sheer sock
short suit
she sat
shoe sack
shy sort
shoe sole
sheet sale
sharp sword
she's sad
short side
sharp suit
sure sign
short sword
shy side
shoe sale
she said
short socks
ship's sail
sharp sound
Shawn's sad

ʃ – tʃ Contrasts

sheep – cheap
sheet – cheat

shin – chin
ship – chip

shock – chalk
shop – chop

shows – chose

shoe – chew
shoes – choose

sheer – cheer
sheered – cheered

share – chair

shore – chore

ʃ_ tʃ_ Phrases

she cheered
show Chuck
she chose

she chewed
should choose
she checked

ship's chart
sharp chin
she charmed

ʃ – dʒ Contrasts

sheen – Jean
sheep – Jeep

shade – jade
shake – Jake
shale – jail
Shane – Jane

shed – Jed
chef – Jeff

shack – Jack
sham - jam

Shawn – John
shot – jot

show – Joe
shown – Joan

shirk – jerk

sheer – jeer

Char – jar

ʃ_ dʒ_ Phrases

show Jeff

sharp jab

shove Jake

ʃ – ð Contrasts

she – thee

show – though
shows – those

share – there
shares – theirs

ʃ__ ð__ Phrases

shut this
shut that
shut these
shut those
shut them
share this
share that
share these
share those
share them

shake this
shake that
shake these
shake those
shake them
shine this
shine that
shine these
shine those
shine them

show this
show that
show these
show those
show them

ʃ – θ Contrasts

shin – thin
shot – thought
shy – thigh

ʃ__ θ__ Phrases

sure thing
she thought

sharp thing
sharp thorn

shy thing
she thinks

Words of Increasing Length and Phrases That Begin with /ʃ/

shade	shady	shadier
shake	shaky	shakier
sharp	sharpen	sharpener
show	showman	showmanship
shame	shameful	shamefully
share	sharecrop	sharecropper
shock	shocking	shockingly
shop	shopping	shopping center
ship	ships	ship's papers
shoot	shooting	shooting star
shark	sharkskin	sharkskin suit

Sentences with /ʃ/

1. Shhhhhhh!
2. He sure is short.
3. She's not bashful.
4. His Chevy is shot.
5. Shape up or ship out!
6. You should show them.
7. I sure am short on cash.
8. Shine your shoes, Mister?
9. She bought some fresh fish.
10. Push the Chevy into the garage.
11. The sun should shine pretty soon.
12. Shake out the sheets on the porch.
13. Be sure to shut the door to the shop.
14. Surely a new leash law is the solution.
15. Does the sideshow have a sharp shooter?
16. You better shine your shoes before the show.
17. She stole the show when she sashayed onto the stage.

t__

tea, teach, teak, teal, team, teen, teeth, tease

tick, Tim, tin, tip

take, tail, tame, tape

Ted, tell, ten

tab, tad, tack, tan, tap

tub, touch, tug, tuck, ton, tongue

Todd, talk, tall, Tom, top, toss, taught

toe, toad, toll, tone, tote, toes

took

two, tube, tool, tomb, tune, toot, tooth

towel

tie, tide, tile, time, type, tight, ties

toy, toil, toys

term, turn

tire, tired, tires

tar, tarp, tart

tore, torch, torque, torn

t__ t__ Phrases

tick-tock	two teeth	type two
take time	tea time	tall talk
top tune	tough talk	two ton
tom-tom	ten ties	two toes
two-tone	tall tale	tin tub
tough time	too tame	tea torte
take ten	top teeth	take turns
tie tack	tell time	two times
too tart	touch tone	ten teeth
top ten	tight tie	tasty treat

__t

eat, beat, cheat, feet, meat, neat, Pete, seat, sheet, wheat

it, bit, fit, hit, kit, lit, mitt, knit, pit, sit, wit

ate, bait, date, fate, gate, hate, Kate, late, mate, rate, wait

bet, get, jet, let, met, net, pet, set, vet, wet, yet

at, bat, chat, fat, hat, cat, mat, gnat, pat, rat, sat, vat

but, gut, hut, cut, mutt, nut, putt, rut, shut, Tut, what

ought, bought, dot, fought, got, hot, jot, cot, lot, knot, pot, rot, shot, taught, thought, yacht

oat, boat, goat, coat, moat, note, wrote, tote, vote

boot, hoot, loot, newt, suit, shoot, toot

out, bout, doubt, gout, pout, route, shout

bite, fight, height, kite, light, might, night, right, sight, tight, white

Burt, hurt, Curt, shirt

art, Bart, chart, dart, heart, cart, part, tart

fort, court, port, short, wart

__t __t Phrases

night beat
cut wheat
cat fight
tight fit
get fat
pet rat
at bat
fat cat
night light
jet set
cut meat
shot put
shoot it
goat cart
white hot
knit hat
nit-wit
get wet
pet cat
doubt it
chit-chat
hot pot
knit suit
putt-putt
tight coat
late vote
shout out

shut it
short note
eat meat
meet fate
heart rate
right height
rat bite
short putt
court date
hurt food
fat feet
neat suit
short sheet
tight shirt
late date
pot shot
tight knot
short chat
thought out
eat trout
wet snout
hot plate
fat trout
brought out
late start
short skit
flat hat

meet Kate
wet coat
sit tight
hot shot
white rat
toot-toot
shout it
white light
curt note
cut out
rat bait
white shirt
meet Pete
bat bite
meet Scott
short skirt
fat brute
sweet tart
spit out
scoot it
best yet
wet paint
sweet treat
right height
white shirt
great sight
plant wheat

t__ __t Phrases

tee-shirt	touch it	tack it
tell it	teen beat	tool set
tea pot	top cat	too fat
top coat	talk right	tune out
too late	take it	tug it
tan suit	too short	tie it
tug boat	time it	type set
tied right	tired feet	turn out
tight fit	top knot	type cast
type it	turn right	top flight
torch light	tight coat	torn skirt
turn it	toy boat	time slot
tight shirt	tease Pete	team sport

t – tʃ Contrasts

teak - cheek
tease - cheese

tick - chick
till - chill
tin - chin
tip - chip

tad - Chad
tap - chap

talk - chalk
top - chop

tug - chug
tuck - Chuck

toes - chose

two - chew

time - chime

tier - cheer

tear - chair

tar - char

tore - chore

t__ tʃ__ Phrases

teak chair	two chairs	torn chair
tall chap	Ted choked	two chimes

t – d Contrasts

tea – Dee
teen – dean

tick – Dick
till – dill
Tim – dim
tip – dip

tale – Dale
tame – dame

Ted – dead
ten – den

tab – dab
tad – dad
tan – Dan

tub – dub
touch – Dutch
tug – dug
tuck – duck
ton – done

talk – dock
tall – doll
taught – dot

toe – doe
toll – Dole

two – due
tool – duel
tomb – doom

tune – dune
twos – dues

towel – dowel
town – down
tout – doubt

tie – die
tide – died
time – dime
ties – dyes

tier – deer

tear – dare

tart – dart

tore – door

t__ d__ Phrases

teak deck
team dues
teach Dick
two days
tease Dave
tin dish
tell Dan
till dawn

talk down
ten days
tan dog
talk down
top dog
took down
too dark
two doors

tuck down
tell Dale
till dark
teak door
teach Dutch
tap down
too deep
take down

t – k Contrasts

tea - key
teen - keen
tease - keys

tick - kick
till - kill
Tim - Kim
tin - kin
tip - Kip

take - cake
tail - kale
tame - came
tape - cape

ten - Ken

tab - cab
tan - can
tap - cap

tub - cub

Todd - cod
tall - call
top - cop
taught - cot

took - cook

toad - code
toll - coal
tone - cone
tote - coat

two - coo
tool - cool

tight - kite

toy - coy
toil - coil

tear - care

tar - car
tarp - carp
tart - cart

tore - core
torn - corn
torte - court

t__ k__ Phrases

tea cup
teach Kate
tin can
tea cake
tin cup
Ted can
tell Kay
ten keys
tan coat
ten cows
top cat

take care
ten cars
toll call
top card
two keys
tool kit
two cars
tight coat
torn cape
tight coil
toy car

torn coat
tan couch
torn kite
teach kids
torn couch
two coins
ten kids
time card
Ted's keys
Todd's corn
trade cars

t – n Contrasts

tea - knee
teal - kneel
tease - knees

tick - Nick
tip - nip

tail - nail

Ted - Ned
tell - Nell

tab - nab
tack - knack

tub - nub

ton - none

Todd - nod
tot - knot

took - nook

two - new
tune - noon

toe - no
toad - node
tote - note
toes - nose

town - noun

tile - Nile
tine - nine
tight - night

toys - noise

tier - near

t__ n__ Phrases

top notch
too nice
two knees
take Nick
top knot

tell Nick
tight noose
take note
teach Ned
take nine

tease Nick
tall niece
teen night
tell Nathan
tell Nancy

t – p Contrasts

tea - pea
teach - peach
teak - peak
teal - peel
tease - peas

tick - pick
till - pill
tin - pin

tail - pale

tech - peck
ten - pen

tad - pad
tack - pack
tan - pan
tang - pang

tub - pub
ton - pun

Todd - pod
tall - Paul
top - pop
tot - pot

toll - poll
taupe - pope
toes - pose

tool - pool

tower - power

tie - pie
tile - pile
type - pipe
ties - pies

terse - purse

tier - peer
tiers - peers

tear - pear

tar - par
tart - part

tore - pour
torte - port

t__ p__ Phrases

take pills
tooth pain
take pause
tan purse

tell Paul
ten pin
tall pine
two pies

take pride
tire pump
tight pants
terrible place

t – s Contrasts

tea - sea
teak - seek
team - seam
teen - seen
tease - seize

tick - sick
till - sill
tin - sin
tip - sip

take - sake
tail - sail
tame - same

Ted - said
tell - sell

tad - sad
tag - sag
tack - sack
tap - sap

tub - sub
touch - such
tongue - sung
ton - son

Todd - sod
talk - sock
tong - song
toss - sauce

toe- sew
toll - sole
tone - sewn

two - sue
tune - soon
toot - suit

tower - sour

tie - sigh
tide - side
tight - sight
ties - size

toy - soy
toil - soil

tier - seer

tore - sore
torte - sort

t__ s__ Phrases

tea set
team song
tin sword
top song
tan suit
ten sows
took sick
top side
take some
too sad
tube sock

tote sack
take sick
tame seal
Tim sat
tease Sam
teach Sue
tin sign
tell Sam
tall sail
turn sign
tong set

torn sail
tall size
torn suit
ten songs
tight suit
take six
two suits
ten seats
take sides
tough steak
track star

tr__

tree, treat, trees	track, trap, trash	true, troop, truce, truth
trick, trim, trip	truck	trowel, trout
tray, trade, trail, train, trace, trait, trays	trough, trot	try, tried, trike, trial, tries
tread	troll	

Words of Increasing Length and Phrases That Begin with /t/

time	timely	timeliness
tab	tabulate	tabulation
taste	tasteful	tastefully
tick	tick-tack	tick-tack-toe
tire	tireless	tirelessly
trust	trustee	trusteeship
tactic	tactical	tactically
terror	terrorize	terrorizing
temper	temperament	temperamental
turn	turnabout	turn-about-face

Sentences with /t/

1. That TV is shot.
2. Take time to talk.
3. Take a turn at bat.
4. This taco is terrible!
5. That Tom. What a nut!
6. He's a teller of tall tales.
7. They went out on a date.
8. Did Tom turn out the light?
9. Tea for two and two for tea.
10. Those two can talk nonstop.
11. That dessert is too tart for me.
12. Our entire team was dead tired.
13. Beg her not to tap dance tonight.
14. I want to eat more but I better not.
15. Take your time eating that hot dog.
16. I wrote a letter to the Senator tonight.
17. You don't need tools to set up the tent.
18. No, Tom, two times two is not twenty-two.
19. It's okay to beat the tom-tom, but not at midnight.
20. We had hot, wet days in September, but not in October.
21. Katie, you can tiptoe through the tulips any time, but please don't do it tonight!

θ__

thief, theme
thick, thin, thing
thatch
thud, thumb
thaw, thought
thigh, thighs
third
thorn

θ__ θ__ Phrases

third thief
third theme
thick thatch
thin thing
thick thumb
three thumbs
three thorns
thirty thieves
think it through

__θ

wreath, sheath, teeth
myth, with
faith
Beth, death
bath, math, path
moth
both
booth, tooth
mouth, south
earth, birth, worth
hearth
fourth, north

__θ __θ Phrases

with faith
south path
both teeth
fourth tooth
north booth
with Beth
north path
fourth moth
north-south

θ – f Contrasts

thin - fin
thought - fought
think - fink

θ__ f__ Phrases

thick fog
third foul
thick fur
third phone
thick fudge
thick fern
thick file
thin face
thick foam

θ – s Contrasts

theme - seem
thick - sick
thin - sin
thing - sing
thumb - some
thaw - saw
thought - sought
thigh - sigh
thighs - size

θ__ s__ Phrases

thick soup
thin sword
third set
think so
thin soup
third seat
theme song
third suit
third sword

__θ – __s Contrasts

myth - miss
Beth - Bess
bath - bass
math - mass
path - pass
moth - moss
mouth - mouse
faith - face
worth - worse
fourth - force

__θ __s Phrases

fourth house
bath house
fourth bus
with Bess
with less
fourth course

θ – ʃ Contrasts

thin - shin	thought - shot	thoughts - shots

θ__ ʃ__ Phrases

thin sheet	thin shell	third shoe
thick sheet	thick shell	third show
third sheet	third shell	three shows

__θ ʃ__ Phrases

bath shop	south shore	north shore

Words of Increasing Length and Phrases That Begin with /θ/

thank	thanks	Thanksgiving
thought	thoughtful	thoughtfully
thick	thicken	thickening
thank	thankful	thankfulness
thorn	thorny	thornier
thirst	thirsty	thirstier
thought	thoughtless	thoughtlessly
think	thinking	thinking cap
third	third base	third baseman
third	third-degree	third-degree burn

ð__

thee, these
this
they, they'd, they'll, they've
them, then
than, that
the
though, those
thou
their, theirs

__ð

teethe
soothe
loathe

ð__ θ__ Phrases

they thought
the thief
their theme
that thick
this thorn
this thick
this thumb
the third
those thorns

ð__ __θ Phrases

the earth
these teeth
that moth
their wreath
this tooth
the south
their hearth
the north
their teeth

ð – v Contrasts

thee - "V"
they'll - veil
than - van
that - vat
thou - vow

ð__ – v__ Phrases

the van	this verse	those votes
this van	that verse	these vines
that van	this view	those vines
their van	that view	they're vain
the vine	those views	their votes
this vine	they vowed	these votes
the vote	their vows	they'll vote

ð – f Contrasts

these - fees	than - fan	their - fair
	that - fat	theirs - fares
they - Faye		
they'd - fade	though - foe	
they'll - fail	those - foes	

ð__ f__ Phrases

they're fat	their food	they found
they fight	this fan	these four
these few	they fit	these five
their farm	their fears	those five
those fees	these fit	their five

ð__ ʃ__ Phrases

the sheep
this sheep
that sheep
those sheep
these sheep
their sheep
the ship
this ship
that ship
their ship
these ships
the sheet
this sheet
that sheet
the shed
this shed
that shed
their shed
the shack
this shack
this shack
that shack
their shack
the shoe
this shoe
that shoe
these shoes
those shoes
their shoes
those ships

v__

veal
Vic
veil, vain, vase
Val, van, vat
Vaughn
vogue, vote
vow, vouch
vial, vine, vise
Vern, verse
veer

__v

Eve, leave, peeve, weave
give, live, sieve
Dave, gave, cave, pave, rave, save, shave, wave
Bev
have, salve
of, dove, love, shove
dove, wove
you've
I've, chive, dive, hive, live
curve, nerve, serve

__v __v Phrases

have nerve
leave Bev
shove Dave
Dave gave
brave Dave
serve Bev

v – b Contrasts

Vic - Bic
vet - bet
veil - bale
vase - base
van - ban
vat - bat
vote - boat
vow - bow
Vern - burn
veer - beer

v – f Contrasts

"V" – fee
veal – feel
van – fan
vat – fat
veil – fail
vase – face
Vaughn – fawn
vile – file
vine – fine
vowel – foul
Vern – fern
veer – fear
veered – feared

__v ð__ Phrases

leave this
leave that
leave them
leave these
leave those
have this
have that
have them
have these
have those
of this
of that
of them
of these
of those

__v __z Phrases

Eve is
Bev is
Dave is
Eve was
Bev was
Dave was
live bees
Eve does
Bev does
Dave does
Eve lies
Bev lies
Dave lies
serve pies
save his
save hers
save ours
save yours
save theirs
give toys
give pies

Words of Increasing Length and Phrases That Begin with /v/

verb	verbal	verbalize
vary	variable	variability
value	valuable	valuables
vacant	vacancy	vacancies
vapor	vaporize	vaporizer
vigor	vigorous	vigorously
valid	validate	validation
vibrate	vibration	vibrations
valentine	valentines	Valentine's Day
veteran	veterans	Veterans Day

Sentences with /v/

1. Give me five.
2. We drove to the river.
3. Very few were invited.
4. Of course he's invited.
5. We will vacation in Venice.
6. Even Faye is not above evil.
7. Chives give it a lot of flavor.
8. Invite everyone to volunteer.
9. He gave his wife a valentine.
10. I crave beef gravy on biscuits.
11. The van was full of valuables.
12. Violets were her favorite flower.
13. He drove his Chevy to Vancouver after all.
14. She was vague about her rendezvous with Victor.
15. The villains have hidden all evidence of their evil deed.
16. Over the river and through the woods to Victor's villa we go.
17. It is not we, why, whoa, wum or vee, vie, voe, vum. It is fee, fie, foe, fum!

w__

In the following section, no distinction is made between /w/ and the aspirated form /hw/.

we, weed, week, wheel, wean, weep, wheat, weave, wheeze
witch, wick, will, whim, win, wing, whip, wish, with, wiz
way, wade, waif, wake, whale, wane, wait, wave, ways
web, wed, wedge, well, when, wet
one, was, what
whoa, woke, woes
watch, wad, walk, wall, wash
wood, wool
wow
why, wide, wife, while, wine, wipe, white, wise
were, word, work, whirl, worse, worth
we're, weird
war, warm, warn, warp, wart
wire
where

w__ w__ Phrases

we won
work week
we'll win
one way
white wine
wide wing
wise word
white wood
we will
which way
we'll walk
worn wood
one wish
weak one
why wait

win one
warm wool
wood wall
wide wedge
we were
wet wall
wise ways
white wall
wet wool
white wig
wise wife
will work
wet one
watch word
warm wind

white wash
one will
wet wood
weak one
we'll wait
one wave
wet wick
we're wise
weave wool
we're well
war wound
wild whim
want one
one worker
walk one mile

w – l Contrasts

we – Lee
weed – lead
weak – leak
wean – lean
weep – leap
weave – leave

wick – lick
win – Lynn
wit – lit

way – lay
wade – laid
wake – lake
Wayne – lane
wait – late

wedge – ledge
when – Len
wet – let

walk – lock

whoa – low

why – lie
wide – lied
wife – life
wine – line
white – light

wear – lair

war – lore
ward – lord

w__ l__ Phrases

we lose
weak leg
worse luck
wet lawn
wise look
we learn
weight loss
wide load

warm lake
wide lane
we'll leave
weigh less
white lamb
wash load
weak laws
white line

what luck
wide line
white light
we lied
one line
white lies
warm light
worst luck

w – r Contrasts

weed – reed
week – reek
wheel – reel
weep – reap

witch – rich
wig – rig
wick – Rick
whim – rim
wing – ring
whip – rip

way – ray
wade – raid
wage – rage
wake – rake

whale – rail
Wayne – rain
wait – rate
ways – raise

wed – red
when – wren

wag – rag
whack – rack
wham – ram

one – run
what – rut

walk – rock
Juan – Ron

woe – row
woes – rose

wow – row

why – rye
wide – ride
wine – Rhine
wipe – ripe
white – right
wise – rise

wear – rare

war – roar

w__ r__ Phrases

we ran
wool rug
well read
wet rug
weight room
wet road
white rose
warm robe
wet rat
we'll race
weak rope

wide row
we're right
wide room
will run
one ride
weak roof
we rode
one rose
wide reach
we're right
wall rack

wet ride
wood rot
one ran
white rock
we'll run
one robe
we're rich
warn Rick
worn rug
wild rose
we raced

w – j Contrasts

whale - Yale

well - yell
when - yen
Wes - yes
wet - yet

whack - yak
wham - yam

Juan - yawn

woke - yoke

woo - you

we're - year

war - your

w__ j__ Phrases

wool yarn
one year

wide yard
weave yarn

white yarn
warm yams

Words of Increasing Length and Phrases That Begin with /w/

week	weekend	weekender
watch	watchful	watchfulness
wed	wedding	wedding day
walk	walking	walking shoes
wait	waiting	waiting room
wash	washed	washed-out
weep	weeping	weeping willow
well	welcome	welcome wagon
wash	washing	washing machine
warm	warm-hearted	warm-heartedness
work	working	working day
waste	wastepaper	wastepaper basket
warrant	warranty	warranty deed

Sentences with /w/

1. We went to town.
2. What a worry wart!
3. Was it worth the wait?
4. Wow! What a windbag!
5. We have a wonderful view.
6. Who will wash the windows?
7. That water was the worst ever!
8. We were given a warm welcome.
9. She gave Walt his walking papers.
10. I always have to watch my weight.
11. Feel that warm wind from the west.
12. Where were you when we went out?
13. I was not awake to witness the event.
14. Will's wife warned him one more time.
15. Wool will hold up well in wet weather.
16. The water is Waterloo, Iowa, is wonderful.
17. I want to wade through the waves in Hawaii.
18. The only wick left was wet and wouldn't light.
19. We were pretty weary after a week of wet weather.
20. He's always there with a witty word when we need one.

/j/__ and /ju/__

Some words in this section contain the glide-vowel combination /ju/ which has similarities to the glide-consonant /j/.

Yale

yell, yen, yep, yes, yet

young

yawn, yacht

yoke

you, you'd, you'll, youth, use

yowl

year

yard, yarn

your, yours

j__ j__ Phrases

your yard	your yacht	yellow yarn
your youth	you're young	You're yellow!

j – h Contrasts

Yale - hail	yak - hack	you - who
yell - hell	yam - ham	you'll - who'll
yen - hen	yum - hum	yard - hard

j__ h__ Phrases

your hair	use half	your hide
young horse	your house	your horse
your heart	use his	your height
yell hard	your hat	your home
your half	young hen	your hand

ʝ – l Contrasts

yes - less
yet - let
yam - lamb
young - lung

yawn - lawn
yacht - lot
you - Lou
use - loose
use - lose

yearn - learn
year - leer
yard - lard
your - lore

ʝ_ l_ Phrases

Yule log
young lad
you're late

young love
you're late
you'll leave

you left
you're losing
you lost

ʝ – r Contrasts

Yale - rail
yen - wren
yak - rack
yam - ram
yap - rap

young - rung
yawn - Ron
yacht - rot
you'd - rude
you'll - rule

youth - Ruth
year - rear
your - roar

ʝ_ r_ Phrases

you're wrong
young wren

yard rake
young rose

your ribs
your ring

ʝ – w Contrasts

Yale - whale
yell - well
yes - Wes
yet - wet

yolk - woke
you - woo
yawn - Juan

year - we're
your - war

j__ w__ Phrases

you win	your watch	you will
your wish	your work	you weren't
young wife	you were	yellow wheat

Words of Increasing Length and Phrases That Begin with /j/

yacht	yachts	yachtsman
youth	youthful	youthfulness
your	yours	yours truly
yank	Yankee	Yankee Doodle
yellow	Yellowstone	Yellowstone Park
yellow	yellowbelly	yellowbellied sapsucker

Sentences with /j/

1. Yes!
2. Yippee!
3. Yes, you!
4. Yes and no.
5. Oh, yes you do.
6. Oh, yes you will.
7. Yes, you know him.
8. You're yellow, Jack!
9. Yes, you can use my ukulele.
10. You're not old, you're young.
11. You're not young, you're old.
12. You need a yard of yellow yarn.

z__

Zee, zeal
zip
zap
zone
zoo
czar

__z

bees, cheese, keys, knees, peas, seize, wheeze
is, fizz, his, Liz
days, phase, gaze, haze, lays, maze, pays, raise, ways
as, has, jazz
buzz, does, fuzz, was
gauze, jaws, cause, pause
chose, doze, hose, nose, pose, rose, sews, shows, toes, those, woes
ooze, choose, dues, whose, lose, shoes
boughs, cows, vows
eyes, buys, dyes, guys, highs, lies, pies, rise, size, ties, thighs, wise
boys, poise, toys
burrs, furs, hers, purrs
ears, cheers, fears, gears, peers, Sears, shears, tears
bears, chairs, fares, hairs, cares, pears, shares, tears, wares
bars, jars, cars, Mars
oars, bores, chores, doors, pores, roars, soars, shores, wars, yours

__z __z Phrases

as is
raise peas
wise guys
his fears
his nose
boys' shoes
raise bees
his eyes
cause fears
his cars
his knees
bee's knees

z – dʒ Contrasts

"Z" - gee
Zen - Jen
Zach - Jack
zone - Joan
czar - jar
zones - Joan's

z – s Contrasts

Zee - see
zeal - seal

zing - sing
zip - sip
Zach - sack
zap - sap

zone - sewn
zoo - Sue

__z s__ Phrases

buzz saw
his soup
lose sight
his seat
was seen
choose some
has soul
choose Sam
lose some
boy's sock
raise some
his sock
gaze south
choose sides
size six

__z __v Phrases

bee's hive
bear's cave
wise Dave
his Chev
choose Dave
his love

Sentences with /z/

1. Who is it?
2. Whose was it?
3. His ears buzzed.
4. That shop is hers.
5. He bruised his knees.
6. His nose is as red as a rose.
7. Flashy ties are not wise buys.
8. These shoes are not size seven.
9. Zach chose not to pay his dues.
10. All she does is sneeze and wheeze.
11. She goes to Joe's café every Tuesday.
12. He has lots of scars from boxing days.
13. Buy these "as is" for seven dollars each.
14. Who knows what those wise guys will do?
15. There's too much cheese sauce on my peas.
16. She always shows her roses at garden shows.
17. His jail cell has bars over the doors and windows.
18. That buzz saw doesn't have the zip it used to have.
19. My fears were realized when the shark's jaws closed.
20. The letter *s* at the ends of words often sounds like a *z*.

3

Vowels and Diphthongs

Most vowels and diphthongs of American English are represented in this speech practice material. Each vowel and diphthong first appears individually in many consonant-vowel-consonant (CVC) words before it is contrasted with other vowels and diphthongs in CVC words composed of similar consonants (minimal pairs). Then it is contrasted with other vowels and diphthongs in phrases and sentences.

DESCRIPTION AND EXAMPLES OF PRACTICE MATERIAL IN THIS CHAPTER

Description of Practice Material for Vowels and Diphthongs	Examples of Practice Material for /i/ as in "beat"
Target vowel or diphthong appears in CVC words with most consonants represented	beach, bead, beef, beak chief, cheek, cheap, cheat deed, deal, dean, deep
Target vowel or diphthong appears in both CVC words in two-word phrases	piece meal weak knees deep sea
Target vowel or diphthong contrasted with other vowels or diphthongs in minimal pairs	bead - bid; bean - bin; beat - bit deed - did; deal - dill; deep - dip heel - hill; heap - hip; heat - hit
Target vowel or diphthong contrasted with other vowels in CVC words in two-word phrases	feed him deep ditch bean hill
Target vowel or diphthong appears frequently in sentences	He has a mean streak. These weeds make me sneeze. Peel the peaches and eat them with cream.

In the practice material presented here, the International Phonetic Alphabet (IPA) symbol for the vowel or diphthong as well a "key word" containing that sound appear at the beginning of each vowel and diphthong section to identify the target sound. Note that a broad phonemic transcription approach is presented in these materials, and the author has taken considerable liberties in clustering certain speech sounds. For example, some vowels and diphthongs are articulated differently in various regions of the United States. The vowel /ɔ/ and its variations are prevalent in the northeastern area of the United States, but it is not as differentiated in mainstream American English where it is more typically articulated as a variant of /ɑ/. The /ɔ/ and variants are grouped and not differentiated here, just as the glide-consonant /j/ and glide-vowel /ju/, as well as others, are not strictly separated.

How can speech practice material for vowels and diphthongs be used in therapy and with what populations?

DISORDER-SPECIFIC APPLICATIONS

Apraxia of Speech or Dysarthria

For people with apraxia of speech or dysarthria, this material may be used to practice a wide variety of speech skills, particularly differentiation among vowels. Most other areas in need of speech practice may be addressed with these stimuli, including prolongation of diphthongs and certain vowels to increase the duration of entire words, reduction of overall speaking rate, syllable-by-syllable production of words and phrases, and improved intelligibility.

Fluency

For people who stutter, concentration on diphthongs and long vowels may be particularly useful for practicing a prolonged-speech technique for fluency.

Glossectomy and Other Head and Neck Cancer Surgeries and Treatments

For people who have had partial or total glossectomy, other head and neck surgeries, and/or chemoradiation treatments to the head and neck that compromise articulatory precision, this material may be used to explore and practice compensatory articulatory gestures, to practice speaking at a reduced rate, and to experiment with pitch and prosodic-temporal variations to enhance intelligibility.

Social or Regional Dialect Modification

For people wishing to modify their specific social or regional dialect, this material may be used to differentiate and practice similar sounding vowels, to change particular aspects of vowels such as reduction of nasal quality, to increase or reduce temporal aspects of vowels (prolongation or clipping), and to modify other prosodic elements in phrases and sentences.

Foreign Accent Modification and American English as a Second Language

For people wishing to reduce their foreign accent and for those learning American English as a second language, the contrasts, phrases, and sentences in this section provide material to practice articulation of vowels and diphthongs, to habituate an optimal speaking rate —usually a reduced rate—to maximize intelligibility, and to practice customary stress-timing-prosodic patterns of these and other phrases that are frequently used in mainstream American English.

EXAMPLES OF GOAL AREAS AND TARGET SKILLS THAT CAN BE ADDRESSED BY MATERIAL IN THIS CHAPTER

Goal Areas	Target Skills
Phonology/Articulation	• articulation of particular vowels and diphthongs • contrasting vowels and diphthongs with each other in word contexts • increased oral openness using long vowels and diphthongs • syllable-by-syllable approach to word and sentence production • overall intelligibility
Rate	• reduce speaking rate by prolonging vowels and diphthongs • increase speaking rate • intelligibility • naturalness
Prosody	• conventional intonational-prosodic patterns in phrases and sentences • fluency and smoothness • syllable-by-syllable production of phrases and polysyllabic words • manner of breathing; breath control • phrasing • naturalness
Fluency	• using a prolonged-speech technique to produce specific sounds, words, phrases and sentences • naturalness
Voice	• increased oral openness using long vowels and diphthongs • best possible voice (free of hoarseness, breathiness, roughness, with appropriate loudness and pitch)

Voice (continued)	• manner of breathing; breath control • phrasing • increased loudness • reduced loudness
Social or Regional Dialect Modification	• articulation of specific vowels and diphthongs that are habitually omitted, substituted, or distorted compared to mainstream American English • inclusion of all syllables of words in phrases and sentences • conventional intonational-stress-prosodic patterns of mainstream American English • intelligibility • naturalness
Foreign Accent Reduction and American English as a Second Language	• articulation of specific vowels and diphthongs of mainstream American English that are habitually substituted, distorted, or omitted • slower speaking rate to maximize intelligibility • conventional intonational-stress-prosodic patterns of mainstream American English • naturalness

SUGGESTIONS FOR USING AND MODIFYING PRACTICE MATERIAL IN THIS CHAPTER

- Use highlighting, underlining, arrows, slashes, and other diacritical markings to indicate the presence of specific vowels and diphthongs, to emphasize them, to indicate pauses, alteration in rate, prolongation, change in loudness, pitch-prosodic variation, and so forth.
- Address one of the client's speech goals, such as sufficient duration of vowels and diphthongs; then, during a subsequent practice of the same material, switch to another of the client's goals, such as intonational-prosodic elements. Later, address both goals simultaneously.
- The clinician may choose to demonstrate a deliberate, slower than customary model and emphasize a particular vowel or diphthong target; for example, to illustrate the jaw, lip, and tongue movement necessary for production of diphthongs.
- Depending on the material, sometimes it is simple for the clinician to add a word to a two-word phrase to make the stimuli only slightly more complex, but less difficult than sentence-length material. Consider adding a word, usually an adjective or pronoun, to two-word phrases as an interim step before moving to sentences.

- Most of the practice material in all sections of this book can be used directly or modified slightly for practice of specific vowel and diphthong targets.
- For additional task variations for contrasting vowels and diphthongs, refer to the Word Grids (Chapter 4) and Contrastive Stress Drills (Chapter 9).
- Self-monitoring and self-critique are fundamental to improving speech skills. Consider recording the client occasionally, then review and analyze the recording with the client.
- Consider using Base-10 Response Forms (Chapter 10) for organizing treatment and scoring and plotting performance of speech management tasks for vowels and diphthongs.
- Delete or modify speech practice material that distracts the client from the goals of therapy.

PRACTICE MATERIAL FOR VOWELS AND DIPHTHONGS

Vowel /i/ as in "beat"

each, eel, eat

bee, beach, bead, beef, beak, beam, bean, beep, beet, bees

chief, cheek, cheap, cheat, cheese

Dee, deed, deal, dean, deep

fee, feed, feel, feet

geese

he, heed, heel, heap, heat, he's

Jean, Jeep

key, keel, keen, keep, Keith, keys

Lee, leech, lead, leaf, league, leak, lean, leap, lease, leash, leave

me, meek, meal, mean, meet

knee, need, kneel, niece, neat, knees

pea, peach, peak, peel, peep, peace, Pete, peeve

reach, reed, reef, reek, reel, ream, reap, wreath

see, seed, siege, seek, seal, seem, seen, seep, cease, seat, seize

she, sheet

tea, teach, teak, team, teen, teeth, tease

theme

thee, these

veal

we, weed, week, wheel, wean, weep, wheat, weave, wheeze

zeal

Phrases with /i/ as in "beat"

piece meal
weak knees
tease me
keep lean
deep sea
knee deep
eat meat
lean meat
each team
neat seam
keep peace
cheap cheese
feed sheep
meet Pete
teen scene
need peace
lean beef
weak tea
pea green
clean feet
sneak peek

real clean
sea breeze
Greek meal
steep peak
green tea
three feet
sweet deal
green wreath
feel grief
clean teeth
green cheese
deep clean
steam heat
green bean
deep sleep
green fee
peach tree
green leaf
deep crease
ski team
clean sheet

sweet tea
deep creek
feel free
green peas
beech tree
keep clean
mean beast
we skied
wheel grease
deep green
leak grease
clean jeans
speak Greek
green sleeve
steam clean
brief speech
clean sweep
sweet dreams
mean streak

Contrasting /i/ as in "beat" with /ɪ/ as in "bit"

each – itch
eel – ill
eat – it

bead – bid
bean – bin
beet – bit

cheek – chick
cheap – chip

deed – did
deal – dill
deem – dim

feel – fill
feet – fit

heed – hid
heel – hill
heap – hip
heat – hit
he's – his

Jean – gin

keep – Kip

lead – lid
leak – lick
lean – Lynn
leap – lip
leave – live

meek – Mick
meal – mill
meet – mitt

neat – knit

peach – pitch
peak – pick
peel – pill
Pete – pit

reach – rich
reed – rid
ream – rim
reap – rip

seed – Sid
seek – sick
seal – sill
seen – sin
seep – sip
seat – sit

sheen – shin
sheep – ship

teak – tick
team – Tim
teen – tin

weak – wick
wheel – will
wean – win
weep – whip
wheat – wit

Phrases with /i/ as in "beat" and /ɪ/ as in "bit"

beat it
keep fit
leave it
each kid

feed it
seed kit
feel it
see it

read it
lead in
steal it

Contrasting /i/ as in "beat" with /eɪ/ as in "bait"

eel - ale
eat - ate

bee - bay
beak - bake
beet - bait
bees - bays

Dee - day
deal - Dale
deem - dame
Dean - Dane

fee - Faye
feed - fade
feel - fail
feet - fate
fees - phase

he - hay
heal - hail
heat - hate
he's - haze

key - Kay
keel - kale
keen - cane
keep - cape

Lee - lay
lead - laid
leak - lake
lean - lane
lease - lace

me - may
meek - make
meal - mail
mean - main
meet - mate

knee - nay
kneel - nail

pea - pay
peel - pail
peace - pace
peas - pays

reed - raid
reek - rake
real - rail

see - say
seek - sake
seal - sale
seem - same
seen - sane

teak - take
team - tame

veal - veil

we - way
weed - wade
week - wake
wheel - whale
wean - Wayne
wheat - wait
weave - wave
wheeze - ways

Phrases with /i/ as in "beat" and /eɪ/ as in "bait"

eat cake
D-Day
deep lake
she ate
keep pace
deep cave
cheese cake
cheap jade

real late
each day
heat gauge
feel great
make tea
main meal
raise beef
league game

safe beach
take heed
same team
raise wheat
same wheel
eight geese
same seat
pay me

Contrasting /i/ as in "beat" and /ɛ/ as in "bet"

each - etch

bead - bed
bean - been
beet - bet

cheek - check
cheat - Chet

deed - dead
deal - Dell
dean - den

feed - fed
feel - fell

geese - guess

heed - head
heel - hell

Jean - Jen

keen - Ken

lead - led
league - leg
lean - Len
lease - less

meal - Mel
mean - men
meet - met

need - Ned
kneel - Nell
neat - net

peak - peck
peep - pep
Pete - pet

reed - red
reek - wreck

seed - said
seal - sell
seat - set

teen - ten

weed - wed
wheel - well
wean - when
wheat - wet

Phrases with /i/ as in "beat" and /ɛ/ as in "bet"

teak deck
real gem
keep them
tea set
deep well
meet them
sea shell

wheel well
beet red
leave them
reach them
eat eggs

tell me

red meat
chess team
bed sheet
red beans
chess piece
red cheek
pet peeve

Contrasting /i/ as in "beat" and /æ/ as in "bat"

eat - at

beach - batch
bead - bad
beak - back
beat - bat

deed - dad
deem - dam
Dean - Dan

feed - fad
feet - fat

geese - gas

heed - had
heat - hat
heave - have

Jean - Jan

keen - can
keep - cap

lead - lad
leaf - laugh
league - lag
leak - lack
leap - lap
lease - lass
leash - lash

meek - Mac
mean - man
meet - mat

neat - gnat

peach - patch
peak - pack
peel - pal
peace - pass
Pete - Pat

reek - rack
ream - ram
reap - wrap
wreath - wrath

seed - sad
seek - sack
seem - Sam
seep - sap
cease - sass
seat - sat

teak - tack
teen - tan

veal - Val

Phrases with /i/ as in "beat" and /æ/ as in "bat"

tea bag
each man
bean bag
feel bad
feed sack
mean man
beach bag
teach math

lean lamb
eat ham

bad deal
gas heat
bad leak
latch key
back seat

bad knee
fat veal
back wheel
trash heap
last meal
grass seed

Sentences with /i/ as in "beat"

1. Peel me a peach.
2. Geese feed on wheat.
3. Lee has a mean streak.
4. Deep sea fish are lean.
5. Does she speak Greek?
6. He was in a deep sleep.
7. Take a sneak peek at Pete.
8. Now he can sleep in peace.
9. They eat beef at every meal.
10. He's going deep sea fishing.
11. Jean returned the key to me.
12. That sea breeze is such a treat.
13. These weeds make me sneeze.
14. Green peas really are pea green.
15. Green tea doesn't agree with me.
16. Clean the green beans in the sink.
17. Don't eat those fuzzy peach peels.
18. The squeaky wheel gets the grease.
19. Steam cleaning will get that grease.
20. Make your speech brief so we can eat.
21. Peel the peaches and eat them with cream.
22. We will freeze our feet without some heat.
23. Beets, peas, and beans again? I want meat!
24. If you eat green cheese, please brush your teeth.
25. He's a Greek Swede who loves eating Chinese food.

Vowel /ɪ/ as in "bit"

itch, if, ill, in, it, is

bib, bid, big, bill, bin, bit

chick, chill, chin, chip

ditch, did, dig, Dick, dill, dim, dip, dish

fib, fig, fill, fin, fish, fit, fizz

gill, give

hitch, hid, hick, hill, him, hip, hiss, hit, his

jig, Jill, gym, gin

lid, lick, limb, Lynn, lip, lit, live, Liz

Mitch, Mick, mill, miss, mitt, myth

Nick, nip, knit

pitch, pig, pick, pill, pin, pit

rib, rich, rid, rig, ridge, Rick, rim, ring, rip

Sid, sick, sill, sin, sing, sip, sis, sit, sieve

shin, ship

tiff, tick, till, Tim, tin, tip

thick, thin, thing

this

Vic

witch, wig, wick, will, whim, win, wing, whip, wish, wit, with, wiz

Phrases with /ɪ/ as in "bit"

give in
chip dip
nit wit
big ship
his wish
this bill
fill in
fish dish
kick it
ill will
dig in
thin chin
hit him
pitch in
win it
big pig
fit in

rich dish
sip it
miss him
big wig
thick rib
fish fin
his gym
thin lip
pick it
king pin
big ring
rich king
king fish
Sing-Sing
wing-ding
his ring
big kiss

wish list
thick skin
dip stick
sick list
stick pin
pin prick
quick dip
skip it
big trip
slim Jim
flip it
hit list
tin grin
skim milk
slick trick
spill milk

Contrasting /ɪ/ as in "bit" with /eɪ/ as in "bait"

ill - ale
it - ate

bib - babe
bill - bale
bit - bait

chin - chain

dill - Dale
dim- dame

fill - fail
fit - fate
fizz - phase

gill - Gayle
give - gave

hill - hail
hit - hate
his - haze

Jill - jail
gin - Jane

kick - cake
kill - kale
kin - cane
Kip - cape
kiss - case
kit - Kate

lid - laid
lick - lake
limb - lame
Lynn - lane
lit - late

Mick - make
mill - mail
miss - mace
mitt - mate

nil - nail

pill - pail
pin - pain

rid - raid
ridge - rage
Rick - rake

sill - sail
sin -sane
sieve - save

shin - Shane
ship - shape

tick - take
till - tail
Tim - tame
tip - tape

wick - wake
will - whale
win - wane
wit - wait

Phrases with /ɪ/ as in "bit" and /eɪ/ as in "bait"

thin veil
in vain
his age
rich cake
fish bait
thin chain
pitch hay

big date
this way
big pain
thin rail
pick names
thick haze
pay bills

make it
jade ring
take it
same wish
save this
take in
they will

Contrasting /ɪ/ as in "bit" with /ɛ/ as in "bet"

itch - etch

bid - bed
big -beg
bill - bell
bin - Ben
bit - bet

chick - check

did -dead
Dick - deck

fill - fell

hid - head
hick - heck
hill - hell

Jill - gel
gym - gem
gin - Jen

lid - led
Lynn - Len
lit - let

mill - Mel
miss - mess
mitt - met

Nick - neck
knit - net

pig - peg
pick - peck
pin - pen
pit - pen

rid - red
Rick - wreck

Sid - said
sill - sell
sit - set

till - tell
tin - ten

will - well
win - when
wit - wet

Phrases with /ɪ/ as in "bit" and /ɛ/ as in "bet"

fish net
big wreck
hit men
ship wreck
big bed
pig pen
Big Ben
thick head
big head
thin shell
rich men
kick them
sick bed
thick neck
get him
ten pin
check him
egg dish
fetch it
tell him
pet pig
sell it
get rich
send him

Contrasting /ɪ/ as in "bit" with /æ/ as in "bat"

ill - Al
in - an
it - at
is - as

bid - bad
big - bag
bin - ban
Bing - bang
bit - bat

did - dad
dim - dam

fin - fan
fit - fat

gig - gag

hitch - hatch
hid - had
him - ham
hit - hat
his - has

Jim - jam
gin - Jan

kin - can
kit - cat

lid - lad
limb - lamb
lip - lap

Mitch - match
Mick - Mac
miss - mass

Nick - knack
nip - nap
knit - gnat

pitch - patch
pick - pack
pill - pal
pin - pan
pit - pat

rig - rag
Rick - rack
rim - ram
rip - rap

Sid - sad
sick - sack
sip - sap
sis - sass
sit - sat
sieve - salve

tick - tack
tin - tan
tip - tap

wick - whack

Phrases with /ɪ/ as in "bit" and /æ/ as in "bat"

give back
big bang
tin can
thin man
big gag
tip back
dish rack
tin badge
chit-chat
his dad

rich man
zig-zag
big fad
sick lad
knick-knack
his back
big bash

hat pin
bad chill

as is
catch it
fat pig
add this
hang him
at will
catch fish
match it
bad fit
pack it

Sentences with /ɪ/ as in "bit"

1. She is still sick.
2. It's a bitter pill.
3. Liz hid it again.
4. Tim is in the gym.
5. Mick did an Irish jig.
6. Dick skinned his knee.
7. Lynn gave Sid a big kiss.
8. Fill it to the rim with skim milk.
9. Tim caught a fish in Chilly River.
10. Living in a big city isn't easy for me.
11. Richard bit his lip when he kissed Liz.
12. Drink skim milk to keep slim and trim.
13. A tick bit Nick in the middle of his chin.
14. Vic packed up his things and hit the road.
15. It calls for a little pin prick on the finger tip.
16. Liz knew him by his thick lips and weak chin.
17. The thief pinned him down and took his billfold.
18. Dick got rid of his old pickup just in the nick of time.
19. Rick grinned, licked his lips, and bit into a big grilled steak.

Diphthong /eɪ/ as in "bait"

Abe, aid, age, ache, ale, aim, ape, ace, ate

bay, babe, beige, bake, bale, base, bait, bathe

chain, chase

day, Dale, dame, Dane, date, Dave, days

Faye, fade, fake, feign, face, fate, phase

Gabe, gauge, Gayle, game, gain, gape, gate, gave, gaze

hay, hail, hate, haze

Jay, jade, Jake, jail, Jane

Kay, cage, cake, kale, came, cane, cape, case, Kate, cave

lay, laid, lake, lame, lane, lace, late, lathe

may, made, make, mail, maim, main, mayor, mace, mate, maze

nail, name

pay, paid, page, pale, pain, pace, pave

ray, raid, rage, rake, rail, rain, race, rate, raise

say, safe, sage, sake, sail, same, sane, save

shade, shake, shale, shame, Shane, shape, shave

take, tail, tame, tape

they

veil, vain, vase

way, wade, waif, wage, wake, whale, Wayne, wave, ways

Phrases with /eɪ/ as in "bait"

they ate	gain fame	stay late
same name	lace veil	Grade A
make way	late date	save space
pay raise	same pace	they stayed
chain gang	lace cape	same place
they came	May Day	great day
ate late	came late	snake cage
pay day	save face	great fame
gain weight	rain gauge	stale cake
late mail	bake sale	main stage
ate cake	Faye's age	great pain
cake bake	same rate	stale ale
name change	beige lace	great shape
late game	main cave	crave cake
same page	gain fame	rain stain
bale hay	hate mail	plain Jane
main gate	make waves	brain wave
same shape	space race	Great Lake

Contrasting /eɪ/ as in "bait" and /aɪ/ as in "bite"

aid – I'd
ache – Ike
ale – I'll
aim – I'm
ace – ice

bay – by
bake – bike
bait – bite

day – die
Dale – dial
Dane – dine
Dave – dive
days – dyes

fate – fight

gaze – guys

hay – high
hate –height

Kate – kite

lay – lie
laid – lied
lake – like
lame – lime
lane – line
lace – lice
late – light

may – my
make – Mike
mail – mile
main – mine
mace – mice
mate – might

nail – Nile
pay – pie
pale – pile
pain – pine

ray – rye
raid – ride
rain – Rhine
race – rice
rate – right

say – sigh
sane – sign

Shane – shine

tail – tile
tame – time
tape – type

veil – vial
vain – vine
vase – vice

way – why
wade – wide
whale – while
Wayne – wine
wait – white
ways – wise

Phrases with /eɪ/ as in "bait" and /aɪ/ as in "bite"

make ice
take time
safe ride
same time
safe side
raise rice
cake knife
bake pies
take mine
safe dive
eight mice
safe height
pale light
same guy
late night
safe hike
aim high
same side
they lie
save lives
take sides
steak knife
my age
nice day
Ice Age
nine days
live bait
right lane
my way
high rate
I'm game
high pay
my fate
I'll say
rice cake
fine lace
ripe grape

Sentences with /eɪ/ as in "bait"

1. Rain, rain, go away.
2. Jane Pane hated her name.
3. Jay didn't pay his own way.
4. Dave lost his way in the cave.
5. The veil didn't hide Renee's face.
6. Monday was a great day for sailing.
7. Dave paid to have his driveway paved.
8. My date with Kate was a great mistake.
9. Ray gave Mae a bracelet on her birthday.
10. I sprained my ankle in the baseball game.
11. Who played the chambermaid in that play?
12. The rain in Spain stays mainly on the plain.
13. What did Dane say about his date with Kay?
14. A great gale blew rain against the window pane.
15. The candidate paid for a full page ad in the paper.
16. With my wage, every pay day comes way too late.
17. His face turned pale when they took Jane off to jail.
18. On Sundays I always hit the hay no later than eight.
19. Shane was out of shape, but he kept pace in the race.
20. I stayed out way too late and now I can't stay awake.
21. The parade came through the main gate of the stadium.
22. To her dismay, Faye's age was displayed on the front page.

Vowel /ɛ/ as in "bet"

Ed, egg

bed, beg, bell, Ben, Bess, bet, Beth, Bev

check, chess

Deb, dead, deaf, deck, death

fetch, fed, fell

guess, get

head, hell, hem, hen

Jed, Jeff, gel, gem, Jess, jet

keg, Ken

led, leg, ledge, Len, less, let

men, mess, mesh, met

Ned, neck, Nell, net

peg, peck, pen, pep, pet

red, wreck, wren

said, sell, set, says

shed, shell, Chev

Ted, tell, ten

them, then

vet

web, wed, wedge, well, when, wet

Phrases with /ɛ/ as in "bet"

sell less
wet head
get them
red bed
well fed
sell them
less mess
deaf men
bed check
red wren
well-well

red gem
left leg
sell bread
send them
dead end
head west
wren nest
best bet
red vest
best guess
mend them

hell's bells
red head
pen set
let them
wet deck
jet set
red neck
wet mess
red hen
check them
best dress

Contrasting /ɛ/ as in "bet" and /æ/ as in "bat"

Ed - add

bed - bad
beg - bag
Ben - ban
bet - bat
Beth - bath

dead - dad
den - Dan

fed - fad

guess - gas

head - had
hell - Hal
hem - ham

gem - jam

Ken - can

led - lad
leg - lag
less - lass

men - man
mess - mass
met - mat

peck - pack
pen - pan
pet - pat

wreck - rack
wren - ran

said - sad
set - sat

ten - tan

vet - vat

Phrases with /ɛ/ as in "bet" and /æ/ as in "bat"

pen pal
sell gas
red rash
check back
pet lamb
dead cat
bell rang
pet rat

less cash
jet lag
get Sam
death trap

bad egg
mad men
wrap them

bad wreck
half dead
catch them
bad check
gas well
back then
brass bell
fan belt

Contrasting /ɛ/ as in "bet" and /ʌ/ as in "but"

bed - bud
beg - bug
Ben - bun
Bess - bus
bet -but

check - Chuck

deck - duck
den - done

guess - Gus
get - gut

hell - hull
hem - hum

jet - jut

leg - lug

mesh - mush
met - mutt

Nell - null
net - nut

peck - puck
pen - pun
pep - pup
pet - putt

wren - run

ten - ton
when - one

Phrases with /ɛ/ as in "bet" and /ʌ/ as in "but"

dead duck
guess what
pet duck
head up

dead bug
well done
sell one
ten tons

one egg
young men
one gem
bunk bed
pup tent

Contrasting /ɛ/ as in "bet" and /eɪ/ as in "bait"

ebb - Abe
Ed - aid

bell - bail
Bess - base
bet - bait

den - Dane

fed - fade

get - gate

hell - hail

led - laid
Len - lane
less - lace
let - late
gel - jail

Ken - cane

men - main
mess - mace
met - mate

Nell - nail

pen - pain

sell - sale

shed - shade
shell - shale

tell - tale

wed - wade
wet - wait

Phrases with /ɛ/ as in "bet" and /eɪ/ as in "bait"

red face
less pay
wet day
shell game
net pay
pen name
well paid
red tape
ten ways
chess game
jet plane
hay shed
lame leg
save them
make beds
take bets
fake gem

Sentences with /ɛ/ as in "bet"

1. Let them eat cake.
2. I get the red checkers.
3. Ed begged for an egg.
4. Ken's new 'Vette is red.
5. Sell the set for ten cents.
6. Ted has plenty of energy.
7. I bet he didn't get a raise.
8. Deb rang the bell for Ted.
9. Help Jeff get the chess set.
10. Dead men seldom complain.
11. The gem was set in a pendant.
12. If I get wet again, you're dead.
13. Ned says his wife hen pecks him.
14. Les fell into bed, dead to the world.
15. Ken and Bette think they're "Jet Set."
16. Don't set the check on the wet bench.
17. Have you fed the hens in the shed yet?
18. The pilot said the jet's engine was dead.
19. They read "The Wreck of the Hesperus."
20. Beverly and Ben met on the edge of town.
21. Jess will get heck for making such a mess.
22. Your best bet is to get a pet that won't wreck the house.

Vowel /æ/ as in "bat"

add, am, Ann, ash, at, as

batch, bad, back, badge, ban, bang, bass, bash, bat, bath

Chad, chat

dab, dad, dam, Dan, dash

fad, fan, fang, fat

gab, gag, gal, gang, gap, gas, gash

hatch, had, half, hag, hack, ham, hang, hash, hat, have, has

jab, jag, Jack, jam, Jan, jazz

cab, catch, cad, calf, can, cap, cash, cat

lab, latch, lad, laugh, lag, lack, lamb, lap, lass

match, mad, Mac, man, map, mass, mash, mat, math

nab, nag, Nan, nap

patch, pad, pack, pal, Pam, pan, pang, pass, pat, path

rag, rack, ram, ran, rang, wrap, rash, rat

sad, sag, sack, Sam, sang, sap, sass, sat, salve

shack

tab, tad, tag, tack, tan, tang, tap

thatch

than, that

Val, van, vat

wag, wham

yak, yam

Phrases with /æ/ as in "bat"

half back
bad rash
hang man
sat back
catch bass
sad sack
fat cat
back pack
gas can
mad man
tap-tap
hat rack
that man
bad gash
sad man
at bat
gas cap
fat lamb
rag bag
pack rat
flat slab
stack cans
last stand

can-can
bad man
tan hat
bath mat
bad back
bang-bang
jazz man
bad pass
fat calf
half bath
ham hash
fat bass
Bat Man
flash back
jazz band
trash bag
gas mask
catch that
last laugh
sand bag
fast track
brass band
flat hand

rat trap
trash man
back track
black cat
at last
grab bag
black hat
bad plan
black lamb
bad crash
fan dance
last man
black calf
brass fan
scat cat
brass plaque
class act
quack-quack
hand slap
crab grass
sand crab
black mask

Contrasting /æ/ as in "bat" with /ʌ/ as in "but"

bad - bud
back - buck
badge - budge
ban - bun
bass - bus
bat - but

dad - dud
dam - dumb
Dan - done

fan - fun

gal - gull
gas - Gus
gash - gush

hatch - hutch
half - huff
hack - Huck
ham - hum
hang - hung
hash - hush
hat - hut

jag - jug

cab - cub
cad - cud
calf - cuff
cap - cup
cat - cut

lag - lug
lack - luck

mad - mud
Mac - muck
mass - muss
mash - mush
mat - mutt

pack - puck
pan - pun
pass - puss
pat - putt

rag - rug
ram - rum
ran - run
rang - rung
rash - rush
rat - rut

sack - suck
Sam - some
sang - sung

tab - tub
tag - tug
tack - tuck
tan - ton

Phrases with /æ/ as in "bat" and /ʌ/ as in "but"

half done
have fun
bad luck
half cup
bad cut
pack up
bath tub
that much

bad pun
half shut
back rub
fat judge
man hunt
half nuts

gun rack

dull tack
run back
cup rack
hub cap
come back
mud bath
young man

Contrasting /æ/ as in "bat" and /ɑ/ as in "pot" or "bought"

add - odd
Al - all
Ann - on

bag - bog

Dan - dawn

fan - fawn
fat - fought

gab - gob
gal - gall

hack - hawk
Hal - hall
hat - hot

cab - cob
calf - cough
Cal - call
can - con
cap - cop
cat - cot

nab - knob
nag - nog
knack - knock

pad - pod
pack - pock
pal - Paul
pan - pawn
pat - pot

rack - rock
ran - Ron
rang - wrong
rat - rot

sad - sod
sang - song
sap - sop
sass - sauce
sat - sought

tad - Todd
tack - talk
tap - top

Phrases with /æ/ as in "bat" and /ɑ/ as in "pot" or "bought"

add on
back off
bad cough
half gone
ham hock
mad dog
sad song

tack on
add sauce
have not
hats off

hot pan
wall map

call back
long nap
wrong man
wash rag
top man
wrong path
watch Sam

Contrasting /æ/ as in "bat" and /eɪ/ as in "bait"

add - aid
am - aim
at - ate

back - bake
bass - base
bat - bait

dam - dame
Dan - Dane

fad - fade
fat - fate

gal - Gayle
gap - gape

hat - hate
has - haze

Jack - Jake
Jan - Jane

can - cane
cap - cape
cat - Kate

lad - laid
lack - lake
lamb - lame
lass - lace

mad - made
Mac - make
man - main
mass - mace
mat - mate

pad - paid
pal - pale
pan - pain
pass - pace

rack - rake
ran - rain
rat - rate

sack - sake
Sam - same

tack - take
tap - tape

van - vain

Phrases with /æ/ as in "bat" and /eɪ/ as in "bait"

back pain
bad name
half page
rat race
gas gauge
back pay

lamb's tail

cake pan
gate pass
they have
same path

mail bag
main match
play catch
grape jam
pay cash

Sentences with /æ/ as in "bat"

1. Catch as catch can.
2. Jack Sprat ate no fat.
3. Put the gas can back.
4. Is her handbag black or tan?
5. We have a cat that catches rats.
6. Take that can of pineapple back.
7. Don't laugh now, but Jack is at bat.
8. Ann is back at the hamburger stand.
9. Dan got rid of the rats as if by magic.
10. There's a rack of old hats in the attic.
11. I'm mad at Pat and want my cash back.
12. The cast thought the last act was fantastic.
13. In January, Chad and Pam went to Atlanta.
14. Sam has a bad rash on the back of his hand.
15. I will have salmon, mashed potatoes, and salad.
16. I'll have a ham salad sandwich and a glass of tea.
17. I asked for a fast Cadillac and I got a sad Pontiac.
18. We will travel the vast lands of Canada and Alaska.
19. Mary had a little lamb, and so did Sandy, Sam, and Dan.

Vowel /ʌ/ as in "but"

of, up, us

bud, buff, bug, budge, buck, bum, bun, bus, but, buzz

chug, Chuck, chum

dud, dug, duck, dull, dumb, done, dove, does

fudge, fun, fuss, fuzz

gum, gun, Gus, gut

hub, huff, hug, hull, hum, hush, hut

jug, judge

cub, cuff, come, cup, cut

lug, luck, lull, lung, lush, love

much, mud, muff, mug, mum, mush, mutt

nub, nudge, null, numb, none, nut

pub, puff, pun, pup, pus, putt

rub, rough, rug, rum, run, rung, rush, rut

sub, such, suck, some, sun, sung

shut, shove

tub, touch, tough, tug, tuck, ton, tongue

thud, thumb

one, what, was

Phrases with /ʌ/ as in "but"

one ton
come up
tough luck
lug nut
some fun
young love
what luck

one cup
shut up
tough one
mud hut
tough judge
numb thumb
what fun

putt-putt
dumb mutt
young blood
hum drum
thumbs up
dump truck

Contrasting /ʌ/ as in "but" and /aʊ/ as in "cow"

bud - bowed
but - bout
buzz - boughs
done - down
gun - gown
gut - gout
hull - howl
nun - noun
putt - pout
rut - route
shut - shout
ton - town

Sentences with /ʌ/ as in "but"

1. My thumb is numb.
2. Did it come undone?
3. Gus has no gumption.
4. This lug nut won't budge.
5. As snug as a bug in a rug.
6. Run up and give her a hug.
7. Shut up, you knuckle head!
8. Does the bus come by here?
9. Come up here and have some.
10. The truck was stuck in the mud.
11. Come up and see me some time.
12. The bus got stuck in a muddy rut.
13. Chuck was stung by the love bug.
14. It's just too much fuss to make fudge.
15. I love to sip a mug of hot buttered rum.
16. The bumblebee buzzed around the rosebud.
17. Chuck's my buddy, but sometimes he's such a chump!
18. Well, dumb-dumb, here's another fine mess you've gotten us into.
19. It was pretty dull being stuck in a submarine one month after another.

Vowel /ɑ/ as in "pot"

In this section, no distinction has been made between the vowel /ɑ/ as in "pot" and /ɔ/ as in "bought." These vowels have very similar pronunciation in some regions of the United States, but the difference is quite marked in others. The material presented here should be altered by the clinician as needed.

odd, off, all, on

baa, Bob, botch, bog, ball, bomb, bop, boss, bought

chalk, chop

dock, dog, dodge, doll, dawn, dot

fog, fall, fawn, fought

gob, gong, gawk, gall, gone, gosh, got, gauze

ha, hog, hawk, hall, hop, hot

jaw, job, jog, John, jot, jaws

cob, cod, cough, call, con, cop, cot, cause

law, lock, log, lodge, lawn, long, loss, lot, laws

ma, mob, mock, mall, mom, mop, moss, moth

knob, notch, nod, knock, not

paw, pod, Paul, pawn, pop, posh, pot, pause

rob, rod, rock, Ron, wrong, Ross, rot

saw, sob, sod, sock, song, sauce, sought

shock, shawl, Shawn, shop, shot

Todd, talk, tall, Tom, tong, top, toss, taught

thaw, thawed, thong, thought

watch, wad, walk, wall, wash

yawn, yacht

Phrases with /ɑ/ as in "pot"

bon-bon
hot shot
rock wall
long song
watch dog
hock shop
long pause
top song
long walk
knock-knock
rock walk
long gone
odd job
shop talk
long call
doll shop
long yawn
drop off
wrong box

top dog
long fall
call off
pawn shop
lock jaw
wrong song
long shot
dog paws
pot shot
top notch
log wall
odd ball
hot sauce
wash off
mop top
box top
clock shop
small pond
swan pond

cross walk
small lawn
lost cause
long stop
small hall
lost ball
swan song
lost watch
small doll
tossed off
small shop
long claws
lost all
small cod
hot stock
small rock
lock box
fall frost
crossed off

Contrasting /ɑ/ as in "pot" and /ʊ/ as in "book"

fall - full
fought - foot
hock - hook
cod - could
lock - look

knock - nook
Paul - pull
posh - push
pot - put
shock - shook

talk - took
wad - wood
wall - wool

Phrases with /ɑ/ as in "pot" and /ʊ/ as in "book"

law book
tall bush
song book
shot put
saw wood
long look
log book

wrong foot
all full
hot foot

took off
put on
shook off

good job
push off
put off
good cause
wool sock

Contrasting /ɑ/ as in "pot" and /ʌ/ as in "but"

bog - bug
bomb - bum

dog - dug
dock - duck
doll - dull
dawn - done

fawn - fun

gone - gun
got - gut

hog - hug
hawk - Huck
hall - hull
hot - hut

jog - jug
jot - jut

cob - cub
cough - cuff
cop - cup
cot - cut

log - lug
lock - luck

mock - muck
mom - mum
moss - muss

knob - nub
not - nut

pock - puck
pawn - pun
pop - pup
pot - putt

rob - rub
Ron - run
wrong - rung
Ross - Russ
rot - rut

talk - tuck
taught - Tut

Phrases with /ɑ/ as in "pot" and /ʌ/ as in "but"

all done
not young
pop up
not one
long putt
wash up
not much

buzz saw
duck walk
come on
tough laws
cut off
rush job
shut off
buzz off

lush lawn
one notch
rough rock
one song
tough talk
bug off
tough job

Contrasting /ɑ/ as in "pot" and /oʊ/ as in "boat"

odd - ode
on - own

ball - bowl
bought - boat

fall - foal
fawn - phone

gall - goal
got - goat

ha - hoe
hall - hole
hop - hope

jaw - Joe
John - Joan

cod - code
call - coal
con - cone
cop - cope
cot - coat

law - low
lawn - loan

ma - mow
mall - mole
mop - mope

not - note

Paul - pole
pop - pope
pause - pose

rob - robe
rod - rode
Ron - roan
rot - wrote

saw - sew
sod - sewed
sock - soak
sop - soap

Todd - toad
tall - toll
taught - tote

Phrases with /ɑ/ as in "pot" and /oʊ/ as in "boat"

long coat
call home
long nose
wall phone
walk home
on loan
not known

gone home
long moan
wrong goal
gall stone

phone call
go on

show off
no socks
roll off
no cause
hose off
mow lawns
doze off

Contrasting /ɑ/ as in "pot" and /aʊ/ as in "out"

ah – ow

baa – bough
ball – bowel
bought – bout

doll – dowel
dawn – down
dot – doubt

fall – foul

gone – gown
got – gout

ha – how
hall – howl

cause – cows

moth – mouth

loss – louse
lot – lout

moss – mouth

Paul – Powell
pot – pout

rot – route

saw - sow
shot – shout

tall – towel

Phrases with /ɑ/ as in "pot" and /aʊ/ as in "out"

long route
pop out
shot down
walk out
log house
doll house

fall down
hot town
jot down
call out
watch out
not now

knock out

foul ball
south hall
loud cough
sour sauce

Contrasting /ɑ/ as in "pot" and /aɪ/ as in "bite"

baa - by
bought - bite

dock - dike
doll - dial
dawn -dine

fall - file
fawn - fine
fought - fight

ha - hi
hawk - hike
hot - height

cot - kite

law - lie
lock - like
lawn - line
loss - lice
lot - light
laws - lies

ma - my
mock - Mike
mall - mile
moss - mice

not - night

pa - pie
Paul - pile
pawn - pine
pop - pipe
pause - pies

rod - ride
Ron - Rhine
Ross - rice
rot - right

saw - sigh
sod - side
sought - sight

Todd - tide
tall - tile
Tom - time
top - type
tot - tight

wad - wide
wall - while

Phrases with /ɑ/ as in "pot" and /aɪ/ as in "bite"

all right
dog fight
long life
tall pine
long hike
on time
wrong size
all mine

all night
long time
wrong side
rock pile
walk by
long sigh
stop sign

bite off
tight wad
guide dog
fine job
dime toss
bike shop
ice box
dive off

Contrasting /ɑ/ as in "pot" and /ɔɪ/ as in "boy"

ball - boil

fall - foil

hall - Hoyle

jaw - joy
John - join

caw - coy
call - coil
con - coin

lawn - loin

pause - poise

raw - Roy
Ross - Royce

saw - soy
Saul - soil

tall - toil

Phrases with /ɑ/ as in "pot" and /ɔɪ/ as "boy"

hot oil
odd noise
top choice
wrong coin
call Roy

wrong choice
all noise
wrong soil
calm voice
pawn coins

soy sauce
coin toss
toy box
loyal dog
boil off

Sentences with /ɑ/ as in "pot"

1. That's a lot of hogwash!
2. Tom is an awful hothead.
3. Don is not cautious enough.
4. That coffee pot is awfully hot.
5. You have got to stop coughing!
6. Ron led the audience in applause.
7. Tom fed the logs into the sawmill.
8. The con man is long gone by now.
9. Their cause suffered an awful loss.
10. Is Tom Small as tall as John Small?
11. Lobster soup costs a lot at the lodge.
12. Tom is awkward and falls down a lot.
13. The fog horn called out from the rock.
14. Connie dropped her shawl on the lawn.
15. The author wants to withdraw his offer.
16. All my calls were to the wrong number.
17. Scott hocked the locket at the pawn shop.
18. The cop caught Tom robbing the pawn shop.
19. Shawn put his calling card by the hall closet.
20. Plans for the caucus were drawn up in August.

Diphthong /oʊ/ as in "boat"

oak, own, oat

bow, bowl, bone, boat, both, bows

choke, chose

dough, dome, dope, dose, dove, doze

foe, folk, foal, foam, phone

go, goal, goat, goes

hoe, hole, home, hope, hose

Joe, joke, Joan

coach, code, Coke, coal, comb, cone, cope, coat, cove

low, load, loaf, loan, loathe

mow, mode, mole, moan

no, gnome, known, note, nose

poach, poke, pole, pose

row, robe, roach, road, roll, roam, rope, wrote, rose

so, sewed, soak, soul, sewn, soap, sews

show, showed, shown

toe, toad, toll, tone, tote, toes

vogue, vote

woke, wove, woes

though, those

Phrases with /oʊ/ as in "boat"

no goal
show boat
vote no
go home
no hope
boat load
Rose Bowl
tow rope
low road
mole hole
ho-ho
no joke
whole loaf
no show
load coal
rode home
whole oats
go slow

soap stone
chrome dome
old crow
coal stove
don't go
no smoke
home grown
Joe Blow
don't choke
slow poke
don't know
go broke
slow boat
drove home
old joke
goal post
oak grove
post hole

stone road
sow oats
snow cone
slow growth
don't smoke
stone cold
so low
stone's throw
nose blow
home loan
rose show
toe bone
boat show
no coal
whole note
road show

Contrasting /oʊ/ as in "boat" and /eɪ/ as in "bait"

oak -ache
oat - ate

bow - bay
bowl - bale
boat - bait

dough - day
dove - Dave
doze - days

foe - Faye
foal - fail
foam - fame
phone - feign

go - gay
goal - Gayle
goat - gate
goes - gaze

hoe - hay
hole - hail
hose - haze

Joe - Jay
joke - Jake
Joel - jail
Joan - Jane

Coke - cake
coal - kale
comb - came
cone - cane
cope - cape
coat - Kate
cove - cave

low - lay
load - laid
loan - lane

mow - may
mode - made
mole - male
moan - main
moat - mate

pole - pail
pose - pays

row - ray
road - raid
roll - rail
roan - rain
wrote - rate
rose - raise

so - say
soak - sake
soul - sale
sewn - sane

shone - Shane

toll - tale

though - they

woke - wake
wove - wave
woes - ways

Phrases with /oʊ/ as in "boat" and /eɪ/ as in "bait"

slow pace
no way
home game
code name
close shave

low pay

lake road
train load
tail bone

race boat
eighth row
make known
take notes
trade show

Contrasting /oʊ/ as in "boat" and /ɔɪ/ as in "boy"

beau - boy
bows - boys

foal - foil

Joe - joy
Joan - join

coal -coil
cone - coin

load - Lloyd
loan - loin

nose - noise

pose - poise

row - Roy
roll - royal

so - soy
soul - soil

toe - toy
toll - toil
toes - toys

Phrases with /oʊ/ as in "boat" and /ɔɪ/ as in "boy"

no joy
road oil
no voice
old boys

no noise
Rolls Royce

royal coach

coil rope
join those
toy boat
coin roll

Sentences with /oʊ/ as in "boat"

1. Oh, no you don't!
2. Joe is such a slow poke.
3. Row, row, row your boat.
4. Joey choked on a doughnut.
5. Go home and phone your folks.
6. Pack your old clothes and get going.
7. I hope those toads don't croak all night.
8. Don't go to the Home Show without me.
9. Put Joan's bathrobe over by her tote bag.
10. Shape the dough into loaves and go home.
11. I wrote my folks to say I'm going to Rome.
12. They told me my trombone solo had no soul.
13. Don't go poking your nose into my notebook!
14. We rowed the boat to Joe's secret fishing hole.
15. The low road was so low we had to row over it.
16. Take a hose to those roses and soak them awhile.
17. With that chrome dome, you don't need to borrow my comb.

Vowel /ʊ/ as in "book"

book, bush
full, foot
good
hood, hoof, hook
could, cook
look
nook
poor, pull, push, put
should, shook
took
wood, wool

Phrases with /ʊ/ as in "book"

good look
book nook
good cook

should look
good push
should cook

good book
should pull
good wood

Contrasting /ʊ/ as in "book" and /ʌ/ as in "but"

book - buck
hoof - huff
hook - Huck

look - luck
put - putt

shook - shuck
took - tuck

Phrases with /ʊ/ as in "book" and /ʌ/ as in "but"

put up
good fudge
wool rug
look tough

good luck
pull up
look young
push up

one book
come look
one foot

Sentences with /ʊ/ as in "book"

1. Put on your hood.
2. He took a good look.
3. The trout took the hook.
4. She shook the rose bush.
5. A wool suit would look good.
6. You should read a good book, Huck.
7. He should have, would have, or could have?
8. Our cook wrote a good cookbook for camping.
9. Don should have looked before he took the wrong turn.
10. You could either push or pull the old wooden door open.

Vowel /u/ as in "boot"

boo, boom, boot, booth, booze

chew, chewed, choose

due, dude, duke, duel, doom, dune, deuce, dues

food, fool

goo, goof, goon, goose

who, hoop, hoot, whose

jewel, June, juice

coo, cool, coop

lube, lewd, Luke, loom, loon, loop, loose, loot, lose

mooch, mood, moon, moose, move

new, nude, noon, noose, news

pooch, pool

rude, roof, rule, room, root

soon, soup, suit

shoe, shoot, shoes

two, tube, tool, tomb, tune, toot, tooth

Phrases with /u/ as in "boot"

new shoes

shoot pool

new tune

toot-toot

new tooth

chew food

two shoes

new rule

cool dude

loose shoes

new roof

loose tooth

cool soup

new suit

blue shoes

two boots

fruit juice

blue room

smooth move

news scoop

too smooth

soup spoon

blue moon

new clue

blue mood

new tools

moose stew

Contrasting /u/ as in "boot" and /ʊ/ as in "book"

fool - full

Luke - look

pool - pull

cooed - could

Phrases with /u/ as in "boot" and /ʊ/ as in "book"

new book
two books
loose hook
rule book

good soup
wool suit
full moon
good mood

pull loose
full loop
cooked goose

Contrasting /u/ as in "boot" and /oʊ/ as in "boat"

boo - beau
boot - boat

choose - chose

due - dough
doom - dome
dues - doze

fool - foal

goo - go

hoop - hope
whose - hose

cooed - code
cool - coal
coop - cope

jewel - Joel
June - Joan

Lou - low
lube - lobe
loom - loam
loon - loan

mood - mode
moon - moan

new - no
nude - node
news - nose

pooch - poach
pool - pole

rude - road
rule - roll
room - roam
root - wrote

Sue - so
soup - soap

shoe - show

two - toe
tool - toll
tune - tone
toot - tote

Phrases with /u/ as in "boot" and /oʊ/ as in "boat"

new boat
two bows
new coat
soup bowl
loose rope
too low
suit coat

cruise boat
blue coat
chew oats

show tune
no room
rose food

cold soup
old goose
don't lose
old news
don't move
cold June
no juice

Contrasting /u/ as in "boot" and /ju/ as in "butte"

boot - butte

food - feud

who - Hugh

whose - Hughes

coo - cue

coot - cute

moo - mute

moot - mute

Pooh - pew

Phrases with /u/ as in "boot" and /ju/ as in "butte"

loose fuse

pool cue

new view

new feud

rude youth

huge shoes

few knew

huge moose

cute pooch

use booze

you fool

Sentences with /u/ as in "boot"

1. How do you do?
2. Have some fruit juice.
3. My loose tooth isn't too painful.
4. Her blue shoes match her new suit.
5. Luann slipped the clue into her shoe.
6. They say doomsday is due very soon.
7. No, Sue bought new shoes, not new boots.
8. The pooch was mooching food from Ruth.
9. Two moose got loose at the Coos Bay Zoo.
10. Did you hear the juicy news about her cruise?
11. The duel meant doom for the new dude in town.
12. Those two could make goo-goo eyes until noon.
13. Luke chews sugar cubes to soothe his sweet tooth.
14. Lou, don't use your soup spoon to eat the goulash!
15. Soon he couldn't loosen the noose around his neck.
16. When you hear "Blue Moon," your blue mood will fade.
17. In the newsroom the rule is "Stay as cool as a cucumber."

Glide-vowel combination /ju/ as in "butte"

The glide-vowel combination /ju/ is quite similar to the glide-consonant /j/. Refer to /j/ in Consonants (Chapter 2) for contrasts, phrases, and sentences with both /j/ and /ju/.

you, you'd, you'll, youth, use

butte

few, feud, fume, fuse

Hugh, huge, Hughes

cue, cube, cute

mew, mule

pew

view

Diphthong /aʊ/ as in "cow"

ouch, out

bough, bowed, bowel, bout

chow

dowel, down, doubt

foul

how, howl, house

cow, couch, cows

loud, louse

mouse, mouth

now, noun

pouch, Powell, power, pout

route

sow, sour, souse, south, sows

shower, shout

towel, town, tout

vow, vouch, vowed, vows

wow

Phrases with /aʊ/ as in "cow"

out loud
cow town
bow out
chow down
loud shout
bow down
foul mouth
down south
shout out
loud howl
gouge out
pow-wow
power house
loud sound
slouch down
brown towel
loud growl
chow hound
round out
brown couch
loud crowd
brown house
found out
crouch down
round mouth
loud grouch
brown cow
round mound
brown trout

Sentences with /aʊ/ as in "cow"

1. Shout out loud.
2. Let's chow down.
3. Now, now, Howard!
4. How now brown cow?
5. The route went downtown.
6. My house is south of town.
7. For crying out loud, sit down!
8. Don't fall down in the shower.
9. Mr. Powell had a bout with gout.
10. Just how did he get out of his vows?
11. Don't go out of this house with that pout!
12. The brown house is further down the route.
13. His loud shout was heard all around the town.
14. There's a mouse in the house under the couch.
15. It's the last brown house on the way out of town.
16. You can take your foot out of your mouth now, Howard.

Diphthong /aɪ/ as in "bite"

eye, I'd, Ike, I'll, I'm ice, eyes, I've
by, bike, bite, buys
chime, chive
die, died, dike, dial, dime, dine, dice, dive, dyes
file, fine, fight
guy, guide
high, hide, hike, height, hive
kite
lie, lied, life, like, Lyle, lime, line, lice, light, live, lies
my, Mike, mile, mime, mine, mice, might
knife, Nile, nine, nice, night
pie, pile, pine, pipe, pies
rye, ride, Rhine, ripe, rice, right, rise
sigh, side, sign, sight, size
shy, shine
tie, tide, tile, time, type, tight, ties
thigh
vice, vial, vine

Phrases with /aɪ/ as in "bite"

high tide
white lie
fine wine
night light
high rise
life line
high time
wise guy
right time
bite size
nice guy
high dive
mile wide
my size
pile high
bye-bye

fine line
wise buy
bike ride
ripe lime
like mine
my side
white mice
I'm fine
nine pies
live wire
by-line
size nine
high sign
white wine
right side
my type

right size
bright eyes
fried rice
blind eye
sky high
night flight
fight crime
nine lives
right price
nice smile
bright shine
slide by
time trial
my style
bright light

Sentences with /aɪ/ as in "bite"

1. I like Ike.
2. Simon has a sly smile.
3. I had the time of my life.
4. If I'd been Ida, I'd have lied.
5. Why not go for a drive tonight?
6. I earned nine titles at the recital.
7. It's a crime to hide an enemy spy.
8. They reside at 119 Riverside Drive.
9. By 1899 the pirates were wiped out.
10. Buy five copies of *Time* and *Life*.
11. It's high time the rivals sat side-by-side.
12. This typing assignment will take all night.
13. Mike bought the fine wine for a high price.
14. The boy smiled as I tied the tail on his kite.
15. I tried with all my might to have a nice time.
16. The bride lied about the size of the diamond.
17. The high bluff is an ideal site for a lighthouse.
18. Diane grows lilacs on the side of her driveway.
19. We finally sighted the plane flying high above us.
20. I'd love to ride side-by-side with you in the moonlight.
21. Ninety percent of the diamond supply comes from his mine.
22. My five-year-old loves the rhyme about the spider and the fly.

Diphthong /ɔɪ/ as in "boy"

oil

boy, Boyd, boil, boys

choice

foil

Hoyle

joy, Joyce, join

coy, coil, coin

loyal, loin

noise

poise

Roy, royal, Royce

soy, soil

toy, toil, toys

voice

Phrases with /ɔɪ/ as in "boy"

boys' toys

boil oil

loyal boy

choice soil

join Roy

coy boy

Sentences with /ɔɪ/ as in "boy"

1. Joyce saves old coins
2. Loud noise annoys me.
3. Put soy sauce on the pork loins.
4. My noisy Rolls Royce needs oil.
5. It was a joy to hear Boyd's voice.
6. The cowboy gave Joy a gold ring.
7. Join the boys and play with the toys.
8. The soybeans were raised in choice soil.

Vowel /ɝ/ and variants as in "burr"

urge, earn, earth

burr, birch, bird, Burke, burn, burp, Bert, birth, burrs

dirt

fur, firm, fern, furs

girl

her, Herb, heard, hurl, hearse, hurt, hers

germ, jerk

curb, Kirk, curl, curse, curt, curve

lurch, learn

merge

nurse, nerve

purr, perch, pearl, perm, purse

sir, search, surf, surge, serve

turf, term, turn

verb, verge, verse

were, word, work, whirl, worm, worse, worth

yearn

Phrases with /ɝ/ and variants as in "burr"

her turn

third word

her work

third girl

worse burn

her purse

third term

her shirt

bird chirp

shirk work

first term

first work

her skirt

first turn

stern nurse

first search

learn first

stir first

stern clerk

Vowel and diphthong /ɪr/ as in "beer"

ear, ears

beer, beard

cheer, cheered, cheers

deer

fear, feared, fierce

gear, gears

here

jeer, jeered, jeers

leer, leered, leers

mere

near

peer, peered, pierce, peers

rear

seer

shear, sheared, shears

tears

veer, veered

we're, weird

Phrases with /ɪr/ as in "beer"

we're here

near tears

we're fierce

near here

sheer fear

near beer

here-here

hear jeers

pierced ears

steer clear

Vowel and diphthong /eɪ/ as in "bear"

air

bare, barrel, bears

chair, chairs

dare, dared, Darrel

fair, fares

hair

care

mare

pair, pears

rare

share, shares

wear, wares

Phrases with /er/ as in "bear"

air fare

fair share

rare bears

bear scare

hair care

fair haired

Vowel and diphthong /ɑr/ as in "bar"

are

arch, ark, arm, art

bar, Barb, barge, bark, Bart, bars

char, charge, charm, chart

dark, darn, dart

far, farm, farce

hard, hark, harm, harp, harsh, heart, hearth

jar, jars

car, card, Carl, carp, cart, carve, cars

lard, large, lark

march, marred, Marge, mark, marsh, mart, Mars

par, parch, park, part

shark, sharp

tar, tarred, tarp, tart

Phrases with /ɑr/ as in "bar"

charge card
large car
barn yard
large barge
park cars
large bar
car part
large jar
card shark
large barn
hard heart
large arch
start cars
large scar
dark star
star chart
darn smart

Vowel and diphthong /or/ as in "bore"

oar, oars

bore, board, born, boars

door, dorm, doors

four, Ford, forge, fork, form, force, fort, fourth

gore, gourd

hoard, horn, horse

core, cord, cork, corn, course, court

lore, lord

more, morn, Morse

norm

pour, porch, poured, pork, pores

roar, roared

sore, sword, sort

shore, short, shores

tore, torch, torque, torn, torte

war, ward, wharf, warm, worn, warp, wart, wars

your, yours

Phrases with /or/ as in "bore"

fourth door

war-horse

pour forth

warm port

your court

north doors

form board

warn George

court door

storm door

store corn

your store

more drawers

four stores

porch door

four more

north shore

more corn

short form

four door

war lord

your horse

short course

more chores

north door

pour more

your source

worn cord

more stores

warm drawers

4

Word Grids

The Word Grids are composed of consonant-vowel-consonant (CVC) words, some CV words, and some words with initial or final consonant clusters. The purpose of the grids is to compare speech sounds in a number of ways. The grids provide many stimuli for probing a client's production of consonants and vowels, to practice a particular speech sound in different words, and to practice words highlighting speech-sound contrasts with differences of place, voice, and manner. The grids can be used with various client populations and for a number of purposes. No particular procedure is prescribed for using them. Each grid has unique features.

GRID I

Grid I displays most of the vowels and diphthongs in American English across the top of the grid. The initial and final consonants of the words on the grid appear at the left margin, and some final sounds are consonant clusters. The initial consonants of the words are in alphabetical order and they mark the various sections of the grid. Across each row, the first and final consonants of each word remain constant, while the vowel or diphthong changes. Down each column, the initial and final consonants of the words change while the vowel or diphthong remains constant.

GRID II

Grid II displays most of the consonants in American English across the top of the grid. Vowels and diphthongs appear at the left margin of the grid, and they mark the various sections. Across each row of the grid, the initial consonant of the word changes while the vowel and final consonant remain the same. All words across a given row rhyme. Down each column, the initial consonant of the words remains constant while the vowel and final consonant change.

GRID III

Grid III displays words with initial consonant clusters <bl>, <br>, <dr>, <gl>, <gr>, <kl>, <kr>, <pl>, and <pr> across the top of the grid. Down each column, the initial consonant cluster of the words remains the same while the vowel and final consonants change. Across each row of words, the initial consonant cluster changes while the vowel and final consonant remain the same. Some word-final consonant clusters are included. All words across a given row rhyme.

GRID IV

Grid IV displays words beginning with consonant clusters <sk>, <sl>, <sm>, <sn>, <sp>, <st>, <sw>, <str>, and <tr> across the top of the grid. The word arrangement is similar to Grid III.

ALL WORD GRIDS

Only fairly common CVC words are included in the Word Grids, with a few exceptions. Some words composed of sounds that are not particularly prevalent in American English are not included on the grids. These include words with /ʒ/; words with initial /θ/, /v/, and /z/; words with vowels /ʊ/ as in "full" and /ɔ/ as in "caught"; and words with regional variants of vowels and diphthongs. Words with /ɚ/ and its variants are randomly represented. When fewer than three common CVC words are present in a particular set of words, (e.g., words beginning with /b/ and ending in /p/) those sets are not included on the Word Grids.

Grid I

	/i/ as in *beet*	/ɪ/ as in *bit*	/eɪ/ as in *bait*	/ɛ/ as in *bet*	/æ/ as in *bat*	/ʌ/ as in *but*	/ɑ/ as in *pot*	/oʊ/ as in *boat*	/u/ as in *boot*	/aʊ/ as in *out*	/aɪ/ as in *bite*
b_	bee		bay					beau	boo	bow	by
b_d	bead	bid		bed	bad	bud			booed	bowed	
b_g		big		beg	bag	bug	bog				
b_k	beak		bake		back	buck					bike
b_l		bill	bale	bell			ball	bowl		bowel	
b_m	beam				bam	bum	bomb		boom		
b_n	bean	bin	bane	Ben	ban	bun		bone	boon		
b_nd				bend	band		bond			bound	bind
b_nz	beans	bins		bends	bands	buns	bonds	bones		bounds	binds
b_s			base	Bess	bass	bus	boss				
b_st	beast		baste	best		bust	bossed	boast	boost		
b_t	beet	bit	bait	bet	bat	but	bought	boat	boot	bout	bite
b_ts	beets	bits	Bates	bets	bats	buts		boats	boots	bouts	bites
b_z	bees		bays			buzz		bows	booze	boughs	buys
ch_k	cheek	chick		check		Chuck	chalk	choke			

continues

Grid I continued

	/i/ as in *beet*	/ɪ/ as in *bit*	/eɪ/ as in *bait*	/ɛ/ as in *bet*	/æ/ as in *bat*	/ʌ/ as in *but*	/ɑ/ as in *pot*	/oʊ/ as in *boat*	/u/ as in *boot*	/aʊ/ as in *out*	/aɪ/ as in *bite*
d_	Dee		day					dough	do	Dow	die
d_d	deed	did		dead	dad	dud			dude		died
d_l	deal	dill	Dale	Dell		dull	doll	Dole	duel	dowel	dial
d_m	deem	dim	Dame		dam	dumb		dome	doom		dime
d_n	dean	din	Dane	den	Dan	done	Don		dune	down	dine
d_t			date	debt			dot	dote		doubt	
dr_p		drip	drape				drop		droop		
f_d	feed		fade	fed	fad				food		
f_l	feel	fill	fail	fell			fall	foal	fool	foul	file
f_n		fin	feign		fan	fun	fawn	phone			fine
f_nd	fiend		feigned	fend	fanned	fund	fond	phoned		found	find
f_t	feet	fit	fate		fat		fought				fight
f_st	feast	fist	faced	fest	fast	fussed				Faust	
fl_t	fleet	flit			flat			float	flute		flight
fr_d	freed			Fred			fraud				fried
fr_t			freight	fret	frat				fruit		fright

g_n			gain			gun	gone		goon	gown	
g_s	geese			guess	gas	Gus			goose		
g_t			gate	get		gut	got	goat		gout	
gr_s	grease		grace		grass			gross		grouse	
gr_t	greet	grit	great							grout	
h_	he		hay				ha	hoe	who	how	high
h_l	heal	hill	hail	hell	Hal	hull	hall	whole		howl	
h_m		him		hem	ham	hum		home	whom		
h_t	heat	hit	hate		hat	hut	hot		hoot		height
h_ts		hits	hates		hats	huts			hoots		heights
h_z	he's	his	haze		has			hose	whose		highs
j_l		Jill	jail	gel				Joel	jewel	jowl	
j_n	Jean	gin	Jane	Jen	Jan		John	Joan	June		
j_nz	jeans		Jane's	Jen's	Jan's		John's	Jones	June's		
k_d		kid			cad	cud	cod	code	cooed		
k_n	keen	kin	cane	Ken	can		con	cone			
k_p	keep	Kip	cape		cap	cup	cop	cope	coop		
k_t		kit	Kate		cat	cut	caught	coat	coot		kite
kl_n	clean				clan			clone		clown	Kline
kr_m	cream				cram	crumb		chrome			crime

continues

Grid I continued

	/i/ as in *beet*	/ɪ/ as in *bit*	/eɪ/ as in *bait*	/ɛ/ as in *bet*	/æ/ as in *bat*	/ʌ/ as in *but*	/ɑ/ as in *pot*	/oʊ/ as in *boat*	/u/ as in *boot*	/aʊ/ as in *out*	/aɪ/ as in *bite*
l_	Lee		lay				law	low	Lou		lie
l_d	lead	lid	laid	led	lad			load	lewd	loud	lied
l_k	leak	lick	lake		lack	luck	lock		Luke		like
l_ks	leaks	licks	lakes		lacks		locks		Luke's		likes
l_m		limb	lame		lamb			loam	loom		lime
l_n	lean	Lyn	lane	Len			lawn	loan	loon		line
l_nz	leans	Lyn's	lanes	lens			lawns	loans	loons		lines
l_p	leap	lip			lap		lop		loop		
l_s	lease		lace	less	lass		loss		loose	louse	lice
l_t		lit	late	let			lot		loot	lout	light
l_z	Lee's	Liz					laws	lows	lose		lies
m_	me		May				ma	mow	moo		my
m_d			made		mad	mud		mowed	mood		
m_k	meek	Mick	make		Mac	muck	mock				Mike
m_l	meal	mill	mail	Mel		mull	mall	mole			mile
m_n	mean		main	men	man			moan	moon		mine
m_s		miss	mace	mess	mass	muss	moss		moose	mouse	mice
m_st		mist		messed	mast	must		most			
m_t	meat	mitt	mate	met	mat	mutt		moat	moot		might

n_	knee		nay				gnaw	no	new	now	
n_n					Nan	none	non-	known	noon	noun	nine
n_t	neat	knit	Nate	net	gnat	nut	not	note	newt		night
p_	pea		pay				paw			pow	pie
p_ch	peach	pitch			patch			poach	pooch	pouch	
p_k	peak	pick		peck	pack	puck		poke			pike
p_l	peel	pill	pail		pal		Paul	pole	pool	Powell	pile
p_n		pin	pain	pen	pan	pun	pawn				pine
p_nz		pins	pains	pens	pans	puns	pawns			pounds	pines
p_p	peep			pep		pup	pop	pope			pipe
p_t	Pete	pit		pet	Pat	putt	pot			pout	
p_ts	Pete's	pits		pets	Pat's	putts	pots			pouts	
p_z	peas		pays	Pez			pause	pose			pies
r_d	read	rid	raid	read			rod	road	rude		ride
r_k	reek	Rick	rake	wreck	rack		rock				
r_m	ream	rim			ram	rum		Rome	room		rhyme
r_p	reap	rip			wrap			rope			ripe
r_t			rate	Rhett	rat	rut	rot	wrote	root	route	right
r_st		wrist	raced	rest		rust		roast	roost		

continues

Grid I continued

	/i/ as in *beet*	/ɪ/ as in *bit*	/eɪ/ as in *bait*	/ɛ/ as in *bet*	/æ/ as in *bat*	/ʌ/ as in *but*	/ɑ/ as in *pot*	/oʊ/ as in *boat*	/u/ as in *boot*	/aʊ/ as in *out*	/aɪ/ as in *bite*
s_k	seek	sick	sake		sack	suck	sock	soak			psych
s_l	seal	sill	sale	sell	Sal			soul			
s_n	scene	sin	sane			sun		sewn	soon		sign
s_p	seep	sip			sap		sop	soap	soup		
s_t	seat	sit		set	sat		sought		suit		sight
s_ts	seats	sits		sets					suits		sights
s_z	sees			says			saws	sews	Sue's	sows	size
sk_l		skill	scale			skull			school	scowl	
st_n			stain		Stan	stun		stone			stein
sh_n	sheen	shin	Shane			shun	Shawn	shown			shine
sh_t	sheet					shut	shot		shoot	shout	
t_k	teak	tick	take	tech	tack	tuck	talk				tyke
t_l	teal	till	tale	tell			tall	toll	tool	towel	tile
t_m	team	Tim	tame				Tom	tome	tomb		time
t_n	teen	tin		ten	tan	ton		tone	tune	town	tine
t_p		tip	tape		tap		top	taupe			type
t_t						Tut	tot	tote	toot	tout	tight
tr_k		trick		trek	track	truck					trike
tr_t	treat		trait				trot			trout	trite

w_d	weed		wade	wed			wad				wide
w_k	week	wick	wake		whack		walk	woke			
w_l	wheel	will	whale	well			wall				while
w_n	wean	win	wane	when		one	wan				wine
w_nd	weaned	wind	waned				wand		wound	wound	whined
w_t	wheat	wit	wait	wet		what					white
w_z	wheeze	wiz	ways			was		woes			wise

Grid II

	/b/	/tʃ/	/d/	/f/	/g/	/h/	/dʒ/	/k/	/l/
/i/	bee		Dee	fee		he		key	Lee
	beach								leach
	bead		deed	feed		heed			lead
	beak	cheek			geek				leak
	bean		dean				Jean	keen	lean
	beep	cheap	deep			heap	Jeep	keep	leap
	beat	cheat		feet		heat			
	bees	cheese		fees		he's		keys	
/ɪ/		chick	Dick			hick		kick	lick
	Bill	chill	dill	fill		hill	Jill	kill	
			dim			him	Jim	Kim	limb
	bin	chin		fin			gin	kin	Lynn
		chip	dip			hip		Kip	lip
	bit			fit		hit		kit	lit
/eɪ/	bay		day	Faye	gay	hay	Jay	Kay	lay
				fade			jade		laid
	bake			fake			Jake	cake	lake
	bale		Dale	fail	Gayle	hail	jail		
			dame	fame	game			came	lame
		chain	Dane		gain		Jane	cane	lane
	base	chase		face				case	lace
	bait		date	fate	gate	hate		Kate	late
	bays		days	phase	gaze	haze		Kay's	lays
/ɛ/	bed		dead	fed		head			led
	bell		Dell	fell		hell	gel		
	Ben		den			hen	Jen	Ken	Len
	Bess	chess			guess		Jess		less
	bet	Chet	debt		get		jet		let

/m/	/n/	/p/	/r/	/s/	/ʃ/	/t/	/ð/	/w/
me	knee	pea		see	she	tea		we
		peach	reach			teach		
	need		read	seed				weed
meek		peak	reek	seek		teak		week
mean				seen	sheen	teen		wean
		peep	reap	seep	sheep			weep
meet	neat	Pete		seat	sheet			wheat
	knees	peas		seize		tease	these	wheeze
Mick	Nick	pick	Rick	sick		tick		wick
mill		pill		sill		till		will
			rim			Tim		whim
		pin		sin	shin	tin		win
	nip	pip	rip	sip	ship	tip		whip
mitt	knit	pit		sit				wit
may		pay	ray	say			they	way
made		paid	raid					wade
make			rake	sake	shake	take		wake
mail	nail	pail	rail	sale	shale	tail	they'll	whale
maim	name			same	shame	tame		
main		pain	rain	sane	Shane			Wayne
mace		pace	race					
mate			rate					wait
maze		pays	raise		chaise			ways
	Ned		red	said	shed	Ted		wed
Mel	Nell			sell	shell	tell		well
men		pen	wren			ten	then	when
mess						Tess		
met	net	pet	Rhett	set				wet

continues

Grid II continued

	/b/	/tʃ/	/d/	/f/	/g/	/h/	/dʒ/	/k/	/l/
/æ/	bad	Chad	dad	fad		had		cad	lad
	back					hack	Jack		lack
	ban		Dan	fan			Jan	can	
		chap			gap			cap	lap
	bass				gas				lass
	bash		dash		gash	hash		cash	lash
	bat	chat		fat		hat		cat	
/ʌ/	bub					hub		cub	
	buff		duff		guff	huff		cuff	
	bum	chum	dumb		gum	hum		come	
	bus			fuss	Gus			cuss	
	but				gut	hut	jut	cut	
/ɑ/							jaw		law
	Bob				gob		job	cob	
					god			cod	
		chalk	dock						lock
	ball		doll	fall	gall	hall		call	
			dawn	fawn			John	con	lawn
	bop	chop				hop		cop	
	boss								loss
			dot		got	hot	jot	cot	lot
/oʊ/	bow		doe	foe	go	hoe	Joe		low
	bode							code	load
		choke		folk			joke	Coke	
	boat				goat			coat	
	bows		doze	foes	goes	hose	Joe's		
/u/	boo	chew	do		goo	who		coo	Lou
	booed	chewed	dude	food			Jude	cooed	lewd

/m/	/n/	/p/	/r/	/s/	/ʃ/	/t/	/ð/	/w/
mad		pad		sad		Tad		
Mac	knack	pack	rack	sack	shack	tack		whack
man	Nan	pan	ran			tan	than	
map	nap		wrap	sap		tap		
mass		pass		sass				
mash	gnash		rash					
mat	gnat	pat	rat	sat			that	
	nub	pub	rub	sub		tub		
muff		puff	rough			tough		
mum	numb		rum	sum				
muss		pus	Russ					
mutt	nut	putt	rut		shut	Tut		what
ma		paw	raw	saw				
mob	knob		rob	sob				
	nod	pod	rod	sod		Todd		
mock	knock		rock	sock	shock	talk		walk
mall		Paul			shawl	tall		wall
	non-		Ron		Sean			
mop		pop			shop	top		
moss			Ross			toss		
	not	pot	rot		shot	tot		
mow	no		row	so	show	toe		whoa
mode			road			toad		
		poke		soak				woke
moat	note		wrote			tote		
mows	nose	pose	rose	sews	shows	toes	those	woes
moo	new			Sue	shoe	two		
mooed	nude		rude	sued				

continues

Grid II continued

	/b/	/tʃ/	/d/	/f/	/g/	/h/	/dʒ/	/k/	/l/
/aʊ/	bow	chow	Dow			how		cow	
/aɪ/	by		die		guy	hi			lie
			dine	fine					line
	bite			fight		height		kite	light
/ɪr/	beer	cheer	dear	fear	gear	here	jeer		
/ɔr/	bore	chore	door	four					

/m/	/n/	/p/	/r/	/s/	/ʃ/	/t/	/ð/	/w/
	now	pow		sow				wow
my		pie	rye	sigh	shy	tie		why
mine	nine	pine	rine	sign	shine			wine
might	night		right	sight		tight		white
mere	near	peer	rear		sheer	tear		we're
more		pour	roar	soar	shore	tore		war

Grid III

	/bl/	/br/	/dr/	/gl/	/gr/	/kl/	/kr/	/pl/	/pr/
/i/	bleach	breach							preach
	bleed	breed			greed		creed	plead	
			dream	gleam			cream		
				glean	green	clean			preen
					greet	cleat	Crete	pleat	
/ɪ/		brim			grim				prim
	blink	brink	drink			clink		plink	
	blip		drip		grip	clip			
/e/					gray	clay		play	pray
	blade	braid		glade	grade			played	prayed
	Blake	break	drake						
	blame					claim			
	Blane	brain	drain		grain		crane	plane	
					great		crate	plate	
	blaze	braise		glaze	graze	clays	craze	plays	praise
/ɛ/	bled	bread	dread						
	blessed	breast	dressed				crest		pressed

/æ/	blab		drab		grab		crab		
	black					clack	crack	plaque	
		Brad		glad	grad	clad		plaid	
		brag	drag				crag		
					gram	clam	cram		
		brass		glass	grass	class	crass		
		brash				clash	crash		
		brat	drat						
	bland	brand		gland	grand			planned	
/ʌ/			drum	glum			crumb	plumb	
		brunch					crunch		
	blunt	brunt			grunt				
/ɑ/	block					clock	crock		
		brawn	drawn						prawn
			drop				crop	plop	prop
				gloss			cross		
	blot	brought				clot		plot	
	blahs	bras	draws			clause			

continues

Grid III continued

	/bl/	/br/	/dr/	/gl/	/gr/	/kl/	/kr/	/pl/	/pr/
/oʊ/	blow			glow	grow		crow		pro
		broke				cloak	croak		
	blown		drone		grown	clone			prone
	blows			glows	grows	close	crows		prose
/u/	blue	brew	drew	glue	grew	clue	crew		
	bloom	broom		gloom	groom			plume	
	blues	bruise				clues	cruise		
/aʊ/						cloud	crowd	plowed	proud
		brown	drown			clown	crown		
			drought		grout	clout	kraut		
/aɪ/	Bly		dry				cry	ply	pry
		bride	dried	glide		Clyde	cried		pride
					grime	climb	crime		prime
	blight	bright						plight	
/er/	blare			glare		Clare			prayer

Grid IV

	/sk/	/sl/	/sm/	/sn/	/sp/	/st/	/sw/	/str/	/tr/
/i/	skied				speed	steed	Swede		
		sleek		sneak	speak			streak	
	scheme					steam		stream	
		sleep				steep	sweep		
	skeet	sleet					sweet	street	treat
/ɪ/	skill				spill	still	swill		trill
	skim	slim					swim		trim
		sling				sting	swing	string	
		slink				stink			
	skip	slip		snip				strip	trip
	skit	slit		snit	spit				
/e/		slay			spay	stay	sway	stray	tray
				snake		steak			
	scale			snail		stale			trail
	skein	slain			Spain	stain		strain	train
	skate	slate				state		straight	trait
/ɛ/		sled			sped				tred
			smell		spell		swell		

continues

Grid IV continued

	/sk/	/sl/	/sm/	/sn/	/sp/	/st/	/sw/	/stɹ/	/tɹ/
/æ/	scab	slab				stab			
		slack	smack	snack		stack			track
	scam	slam			Spam		swam		tram
	scanned				spanned	stand		strand	
		slap		snap				strap	trap
	scat	slat			spat	stat			
/ʌ/		slug	smug	snug					
	scum	slum					swum	strum	
/ɑ/		slob		snob			swab		
			smock		Spock	stock			
		slop				stop	swap		
	Scott	slot		snot	spot		swat		trot
/oʊ/			smoke		spoke	stoke		stroke	
	scone	Sloan				stone			
/u/		slew				stew			true
					spoon		swoon	strewn	
	scoop	sloop		snoop		stoop	swoop		troop
	scoot			snoot					
/aʊ/	scout			snout	spout	stout			trout

/aɪ/	sky	sly			spy	sty			try
		slide		snide	spied			stride	tried
			smile			stile			trial
					spine	stein	swine		
		slight	smite		spite				trite
/ɚ/		slur			spur	stir			
/or/	score		s'more	snore	spore	store	swore		
/ɪr/			smear	sneer	spear	steer			
/ɑr/	scar				spar	star			
/er/	scare			snare	spare	stare	swear		

5

Common Expressions

In American English, some expressions are used frequently in everyday conversation. We say many of them without much thinking, and they play an important part in how we communicate. Unlike overlearned or memorized passages such as rhymes and poems or seriatim speech, such as counting, these expressions have purpose and meaning in conversation, as well as an automatic-reactive nature about them. Common expressions are very useful and serve many roles. We say them, or slight variations of them, to initiate, to respond, and to contribute to conversational flow. They are rich material for speech and language therapy.

The common expressions provided here are loosely arranged by length and not by frequency of use because usage varies greatly from one person to another and from one community or region to another. Punctuation other than question marks and some exclamation marks have been omitted to encourage various prosodic patterns and different production styles to convey different meanings. Many of the expressions are obvious and require no context or setup by the clinician, although this varies depending on the expression and the client. Of note is that many common expressions are produced rapidly. This natural and rapid delivery of common expressions can be very challenging when the person with a speech disorder must reduce speaking rate to execute precise articulatory movements for maximum intelligibility.

How can common expressions be used in therapy and with what populations?

DISORDER-SPECIFIC APPLICATIONS

Apraxia of Speech

For people with apraxia of speech, common expressions may be used to practice articulatory gestures, rate, and the timing-rhythm-melody aspects of prosody for optimal intelligibility and naturalness. In addition, practicing common expressions may have therapeutic application to those who have aphasia or other cognitive impairments that often accompany motor speech disorders.

Dysarthria

For people with dysarthria, common expressions can be utilized in many ways, such as to increase articulatory precision, to reduce or increase speaking rate, to increase loudness, to coordinate breathing and phrasing, to practice elements of prosody, and to increase oral openness when speaking.

Voice

For people with hyperfunctional voice disorders who have achieved target voice production in seriatim and overlearned speech, the short and frequently used expressions in this section may be applicable for practicing "best voice" before progressing to longer utterances of more purposive and conversational nature.

Fluency

For people who stutter, common expressions may be well suited for practicing fluency techniques and gaining success and confidence in simulated conversation practice because of their high rate of occurrence and applicability in everyday settings.

Laryngectomy

For people who have had total laryngectomy who use an artificial larynx device, a tracheoesophageal voice prosthesis, or use esophageal voice, and for those who have had other laryngeal surgeries, common expressions may be helpful for working on coordinating breathing and phrasing, improved articulatory precision, timing and pacing, increased oral openness while speaking, as well as for addressing loudness and voice quality.

Glossectomy and Other Head and Neck Cancer Surgeries and Treatments

For people who have had partial or total glossectomy, other head and neck surgeries, and/or chemo-radiation treatments to the head and neck that compromise strength, range of motion, and articulatory precision, these phrases may be used to explore and practice compensatory articulatory gestures, to practice speaking at a reduced rate, and to experiment with pitch and prosodic variations to enhance intelligibility.

Social or Regional Dialect Modification

For people wishing to modify their specific social or regional dialect, common expressions may be used to address any aspect of consonant, vowel, and syllable production, and customary prosody of mainstream American English.

Foreign Accent Reduction and American English as a Second Language

For people wishing to reduce their foreign accent, as well as for those learning American English as a second language, common expressions are an important element of carrying on a conversation. The phrases and sentences in this section provide material to practice articulation of specific sounds, to utilize an optimal speaking rate to maximize intelligibility, to practice customary stress and prosodic patterns in well-known phrases, to learn and practice subtleties and nuances of tone and timing of delivery, and to become familiar with other pragmatic aspects of common expressions essential for their use in American English conversation.

EXAMPLES OF GOAL AREAS AND SPECIFIC TARGETS THAT CAN BE ADDRESSED BY COMMON EXPRESSIONS

Goal Areas	Target Skills
Articulation/Phonology	• specific phonemes in various word positions • consonant clusters and sound blending • polysyllabic words • overall intelligibility
Rate	• reduced speaking rate • increased speaking rate • intelligibility • naturalness
Prosody	• general intonational-prosodic patterns of common statements, comments, questions, interjections, and exclamations • affected style and prosody for humor, sarcasm, inference, etc. • syllable-by-syllable production of phrases • conventional stress patterns in polysyllabic words • fluency and smoothness • phrasing • breath support, manner of breathing • naturalness
Fluency	• using a prolonged-speech technique to produce specific sounds, words, phrases in imitation, oral reading, and simulated conversations • fluent production of common conversational utterances • naturalness
Voice	• variability in pitch and loudness; intonation • increased loudness • reduced loudness • best possible voice (free of hoarseness, breathiness, and roughness with appropriate pitch and loudness) • phrasing • breath support, manner of breathing

Conversational Skills	• rules of conversation; when, where, and how common expressions are used; appropriateness • conversational turn-taking; speaker-listener roles • elements of timing that influence meaning • initiating • responding • commenting • interjecting • quantity of discourse—abbreviating or elaborating • interrupting; overlapping • naturalness
Social or Regional Dialect Modification	• articulation of specific speech sounds that are habitually omitted, substituted, or distorted • inclusion of all syllables of words • customary intonational-prosodic patterns of mainstream American English • naturalness
Foreign Accent Reduction and American English as a Second Language	• slower speaking rate to maximize intelligibility • articulation of specific speech sounds of American English that are habitually substituted, distorted, or omitted • customary intonational-prosodic patterns of mainstream American English • stress patterns of common polysyllabic words • how intonation can change the meaning of words or entire expressions • learning and practicing elements of casual American English conversation

SUGGESTIONS FOR USING AND MODIFYING THE PRACTICE MATERIAL IN COMMON EXPRESSIONS

- Use highlighting, underlining, arrows, slashes, and other diacritical markings to indicate the presence of specific phonemes, to mark syllable separation, to emphasize/stress specific elements, to indicate pauses, alteration in rate, prolongation, change in loudness, pitch-prosodic variation, and so forth.
- Address one of the client's speech goals, such as increased intonational variation or articulatory precision, during early practice sessions, then switch to another of the client's goals, such as naturalness, during a subsequent practice of the same expressions. Later, address both goals simultaneously.
- Practice the material in this section more than once and with different prosodic patterns or styles of delivery.
- In everyday conversations we generally say common expressions quite rapidly. "Quick delivery" is a component of both casual and formal conversations. Adult clients with acquired speech and language disorders often complain that they cannot "jump into" conversations like they did in the past. Yet, the client may need to practice a deliberate, slower than normal pace to emphasize a speech target, such as precise articulatory gestures or a syllable-by-syllable prosodic style, to improve intelligibility. Afterward, and depending on many variables, the task may change to speeding-up certain utterances to make them sound more natural and spontaneous.
- Self-monitoring and self-critique are fundamental to improving speech and language skills. A tried-and-true therapy activity is to audio- or video-record the client saying these expressions. Afterward, the clinician and client review the recording and analyze the speech performance.
- To extend and vary the use of this practice material, the speech-language pathologist and client may think of possible antecedent or follow-up comments to a given expression.
- Variations of therapeutic tasks and the practice material presented here are encouraged if they complement the intended goals of therapy and capture the client's attention and participation.
- Individuals, families, and populations in certain geographic areas have their own versions of these and similar expressions. The clinician and client may use the form, "Practice Your Own Common Expressions" on the last page of this chapter to list and practice expressions that pertain to the client's life, and communication style, partners, and community.
- If the client has the speech and language prerequisites, consider presenting these stimuli in a question-answer format of a Contrastive Stress Drill. See Chapter 9.
- Delete or modify material that distracts the client from the goals of therapy.

PRACTICE MATERIAL FOR COMMON EXPRESSIONS

1. Hi
2. Yes
3. No
4. Hey
5. Hello
6. Well, . . .
7. I win
8. Good-bye
9. Oops!
10. So-so
11. I'll bet
12. I agree
13. Beat it
14. Oh, no
15. No, Sir
16. Sit still
17. Pay up
18. Drop it
19. Oh, my
20. It's hot
21. Be still
22. Keep it
23. Not bad
24. Get lost
25. Stop it
26. I'm fine
27. No way
28. Too bad
29. Let's go
30. Call 911
31. Nice job
32. Just fine
33. Too late
34. Go home
35. You bet
36. Skip it
37. My turn
38. Come in
39. Look out
40. Oh, boy
41. Hold it
42. Stand up
43. You win
44. Dear me
45. Wake up
46. I'm tired
47. Good job
48. You first
49. Watch it
50. I'm cold
51. That's it
52. Be good
53. I'm okay
54. Time out
55. Oh, yeah
56. Cheer up
57. Let's eat
58. Have fun
59. Come on
60. Go away
61. No doubt
62. Beats me
63. Speak up
64. Not now
65. I'm busy
66. Let's talk

67. Afraid so
68. Heads up
69. I hope so
70. Sit down
71. I'm sorry
72. I doubt it
73. Got to go
74. Take five
75. I'm home
76. After you
77. Allow me
78. Why not?
79. Don't ask
80. Oh, please . . .
81. Is that so?
82. I feel sick
83. Keep cool
84. Dream on
85. Go ahead
86. Sometime
87. Cut it out
88. Where to?
89. Let's talk
90. Call again
91. Get going
92. Oh, yeah?
93. Be careful
94. I hope not
95. Afraid not
96. Not much
97. Don't quit
98. Got to run
99. Say what?
100. That hurts
101. Don't slip
102. Not likely
103. Your turn
104. What of it?
105. You wish
106. Sure thing
107. Well done
108. Keep busy
109. It's on me
110. No chance
111. Step aside
112. You drive
113. That's nice
114. Checkmate
115. Soup's on!
116. Try harder
117. Stay tuned
118. Fat chance
119. Is that so
120. Just watch
121. Nice going
122. Very good
123. Fancy that
124. Grab a bite
125. What is it?
126. Don't look
127. Good grief
128. Watch out
129. I'll be back
130. Turn it off
131. You know. . .
132. Excuse me
133. Break it up
134. Put it there
135. Time to go
136. It's for you

137. Keep quiet
138. Your move
139. Good luck!
140. Who cares?
141. You decide
142. Say "when"
143. What now?
144. Yes, ma'am
145. No problem
146. Good grief
147. Guess what?
148. Slow down
149. What if . . .
150. If you insist
151. How much?
152. Good night
153. That's cool
154. If you want
155. That's okay
156. No kidding
157. What time?
158. Ladies first
159. Go to sleep
160. Guess again
161. Which way?
162. Wait for me
163. Since when?
164. My pleasure
165. Don't leave
166. You called?
167. I'm starved
168. Don't argue
169. Where is it?
170. I don't care
171. Break a leg
172. What's up?
173. Turn around
174. Don't say it
175. Easy does it
176. I feel better
177. That's right
178. Good news
179. Deal with it
180. I can't do it
181. Lots of luck
182. Take it easy
183. That does it
184. Neither do I
185. I believe so
186. It's too late
187. Never mind
188. What's up?
189. I'm freezing
190. I don't get it
191. Have a chair
192. Say no more
193. Listen to me
194. Who knows?
195. I'm afraid so
196. Don't get up
197. See you later
198. What's new?
199. I kid you not
200. Where am I?
201. Hear me out
202. I don't know
203. Don't bother
204. I'm with you
205. Not a chance
206. Call me later

207. Take a break
208. I can't find it
209. You can, too
210. That's funny
211. He's a goner
212. Turn on the TV
213. So far so good
214. It works for me
215. Truth be told . . .
216. It's too early
217. Get over it!
218. Hold on there
219. I promise you
220. Check, please
221. Help yourself
222. You don't say
223. Next question
224. Here's to you
225. I can't help it
226. Don't give up
227. Just a minute
228. See you soon
229. There you go
230. Say "cheese"
231. How are you?
232. Good for you
233. What is that?
234. Don't ask me
235. Feeling okay?
236. Take your pick
237. Wait a minute
238. Come right in
239. No, thank you
240. It's time to go
241. Use your head
242. That's terrible
243. I don't want it
244. In my opinion . . .
245. Nothing doing
246. Can you hold?
247. Live and learn
248. Good for you
249. Do you mind?
250. That's enough
251. Who said that?
252. Don't push me
253. Use your head
254. No harm done
255. Good morning
256. What about it?
257. I need a doctor
258. Take the stairs
259. In other words
260. Just you watch
261. I haven't a clue
262. Anything else?
263. That's not fair!
264. Care to dance?
265. I almost lost it
266. Don't mind me
267. What's wrong?
268. I don't think so
269. One more thing
270. Make it snappy
271. I can top that
272. Just wonder
273. Catch you later
274. Please sit down
275. It's about time
276. I'm not kidding

277. Go climb a tree
278. I've seen worse
279. Don't look now
280. Mum's the word
281. Ready to order?
282. Where are you?
283. It's a no-brainer
284. I don't want any
285. Turn off the TV
286. Anyone I know?
287. It's beyond me
288. Don't be so sure
289. Happy Birthday
290. I can't talk now
291. Have a safe trip
292. Leave me alone
293. That's too much
294. Drop everything
295. To some degree
296. Well, excuse me
297. It's a lost cause
298. Without a doubt
299. May I help you?
300. Believe it or not
301. I had no choice
302. You can have it
303. I'm on his side
304. Had a nice time
305. Come back later
306. Run for your life
307. You know what?
308. Glad to meet you
309. My car won't start
310. Like I was saying
311. Don't kid yourself
312. I can't hear you
313. Don't quit trying
314. Come and get it
315. And away we go
316. I have to go now
317. Take it with you
318. Drop the subject
319. You're too much
320. I'm fine, thanks
321. Dinner is served
322. What time is it?
323. Turn at the light
324. What's cooking?
325. Look who's here
326. I spoke too soon
327. Do you read me?
328. Well, for starters . . .
329. Beg your pardon?
330. Don't be so sure
331. How old are you?
332. I need some sleep
333. Long time no see
334. Don't tell anyone
335. You're the doctor
336. Glad to meet you
337. Don't you know?
338. Drop in sometime
339. See you tomorrow
340. May we join you?
341. Answer the phone
342. Forgive and forget
343. If you ask me . . .
344. Get the message?
345. I'm feeling better
346. Keep your chin up

347. You make me sick
348. Give me a break!
349. Call an ambulance
350. What did you say?
351. Don't do anything
352. It could be worse
353. How's the family?
354. You're telling me
355. Because I said so!
356. It's now or never
357. All systems are go
358. Take smaller bites
359. Where's the fire?
360. You don't get it
361. Let's call it a day
362. Well, in that case . . .
363. I'll get right on it
364. I don't like those
365. I'm glad to hear it
366. Not by a long shot
367. I just can't help it
368. Keep your shirt on
369. I can't accept that
370. Better hit the road
371. Let's talk about it
372. I'm sorry I asked
373. What's happening?
374. Keep out of trouble
375. What's that noise?
376. You can't beat that
377. Let's call it a night
378. I'm stuck in traffic
379. How do you know?
380. Who's at the door?
381. Don't let me down
382. Would you please?
383. I'm back on track
384. What do you want?
385. That's the way it is
386. Keep quiet about it
387. I'd like some water
388. At the present time
389. Bite your tongue
390. I don't mean maybe
391. Wish you were here
392. Where do you live?
393. I changed my mind
394. Eat your vegetables
395. Good talking to you
396. It stands to reason
397. Get out of my way
398. Don't forget to write
399. I believe we've met
400. I haven't got all day
401. It's marginal at best
402. Did you lock the door?
403. To be perfectly honest
404. Tell me another one
405. It's anyone's guess
406. Don't get me wrong
407. I can't find my keys
408. How is the weather?
409. Make up your mind!
410. Score one for me
411. Your place or mine?
412. Let's leave it that way
413. I'm glad you told me
414. What's the problem?
415. Look who's talking
416. It doesn't make sense

417. You can say that again
418. Let's get out of here
419. Please pass the bread
420. I'll be right with you
421. Thanks, but no thanks
422. What do you mean?
423. I laughed 'til I cried
424. Let the buyer beware
425. I wish I had said that
426. Better luck next time
427. That beats everything
428. I know them by heart
429. Thank you very much
430. Then what happened?
431. Don't waste your time
432. I've never been better
433. Cold enough for you?
434. I can't say that I do
435. Which way did he go?
436. Oh, for crying out loud
437. Get your act together
438. I'll talk with you soon
439. We've run out of time
440. Things could be better
441. What's going on here?
442. I can't argue with that
443. Where are you going?
444. In my humble opinion
445. We must do this again
446. I'm not following you
447. Where's the restroom?
448. That's another matter
449. If that doesn't beat all!
450. That's hard to believe
451. It goes without saying
452. Do you have the time?
453. I couldn't ask for more
454. I'm not finished with it
455. Can you keep a secret?
456. You can't win them all
457. My house is your house
458. The check's in the mail
459. Did you hear the news?
460. Follow in his footsteps
461. Don't quit your day job
462. Where should we meet?
463. That's not good enough
464. Which one do you like?
465. It's no laughing matter
466. Not in a thousand years
467. That's pretty far fetched
468. Don't hold your breath
469. When will you be back?
470. Wouldn't you know it
471. It caught me off guard
472. It's far from being over
473. That's one way to put it
474. We're going nowhere fast
475. I hear what you're saying
476. We've come to a dead end
477. Times sure have changed
478. Let's shake things up a bit
479. I have better things to do
480. You're missing the point
481. Just between you and me . . .
482. This may come as a shock
483. Contrary to popular belief . . .
484. Everything went smoothly
485. That's easier said than done
486. You could have fooled me

487. Nice weather we're having
488. Just sign on the dotted line
489. I would jump at the chance
490. It's as simple as child's play
491. That's his greatest weakness
492. I'm very disappointed
493. Stop blaming yourself
494. Win a few, lose a few
495. I'm thinking out loud
496. It's not quite that simple
497. Smile when you say that
498. It just goes to show you . . .
499. It isn't worth the trouble
500. I can't thank you enough
501. You know what they say
502. May I have more please?
503. I hate to eat and run, but . . .
504. Well, what do you know
505. I'm delighted to meet you
506. Let's get something to eat
507. I laughed like all get out
508. It's an old-fashioned idea
509. I'm not finished with you
510. I'll see you in a little while
511. There's no place like home
512. I'm on the road to recovery
513. That's the last thing we need
514. I just can't keep them in line
515. That didn't go over so well
516. It was relatively uneventful
517. Thank you for a lovely time
518. I was scared out of my wits
519. That's just wishful thinking
520. And, to make matters worse
521. I hear you loud and clear
522. If you can't beat 'em, join 'em
523. That's a frightening thought
524. I laugh in the face of danger
525. I would do it all over again
526. That's only part of the story
527. Your secret is safe with me
528. We've all got to go sometime
529. That's a little hard to believe
530. You'll be the death of me yet
531. By no stretch of the imagination
532. Thank you for a wonderful time
533. Tell me something I don't know
534. There's a method to his madness
535. You might be able to pull it off
536. Everything but the kitchen sink
537. Truer words were never spoken
538. Things went from bad to worse
539. It has opened up new possibilities
540. Do you expect me to believe that?
541. We've got to start somewhere
542. It strikes fear in the hearts of men
543. You're saying all the right things
544. Perhaps now he'll think twice before . . .
545. I'll do it when I'm good and ready
546. He's the spitting image of his father
547. Have you taken leave of your senses?
548. We made it home safe and sound
549. I've told you time and time again
550. And who can blame him for doing it?
551. But there are some serious drawbacks
552. Sit down and take a load off your feet
553. So, what are you going to do about it?
554. You can take all the time in the world
555. Haven't I seen you somewhere before?
556. Who could have imagined such a thing?

557. It was bound to happen sooner or later
558. If at first you don't succeed, try try again
559. He's gone above and beyond the call of duty
560. It was destroyed virtually beyond recognition
561. He hmm-ed and hawed so long, I finally gave up

"PRACTICE YOUR OWN COMMON EXPRESSIONS" FORM

Make a list of common expressions you say or that others say in your family or community. Then practice them. Tell yourself, "When I say these, I will keep this speech goal in mind"

Goal: ______________________________

____

1. ______________________________

2. ______________________________

3. ______________________________

4. ______________________________

5. ______________________________

6. ______________________________

7. ______________________________

8. ______________________________

9. ______________________________

10. ______________________________

6

Figurative Expressions

In American English, it is second nature to use figurative expressions in daily conversations. The speech practice material in Figurative Expressions differs from those in Common Expressions only in that the familiar phrases and sentences are more abstract or figurative or idiomatic or metaphoric. Indeed, the figurative expressions presented here are very common. Many contain idioms—expressions with meaning that cannot be determined by the meanings of their individual words. Some are clichés—trite, stereotyped expressions. Others are proverbs or adages—sayings that express a commonplace truth or useful thought. The figurative expressions that appear here can be overheard in everyday conversations, heard on television and radio, and read in newspapers and magazines. They are very familiar to adults and to most older children.

Near the end of the figurative expressions in this chapter is a selection of limericks. Limericks are simple, five-line poems that are humorous and sometimes quite silly. Most limericks use figurative language and many are known to have bawdy content. The limericks here have appropriate humor and have been included because they contain figurative language and "plays on words." All can be recited with a predictable and exaggerated cadence and prosody that can be used to address certain therapy goals.

Figurative expressions can be rich material for speech and language therapy. As with automatic speech and common expressions, the familiarity of these figurative expressions may "lighten" language and cognitive demands, making them easier for a speaker to produce than other purposive, conversational speech. At the same time, many figurative expressions are not as versatile and modifiable as are other speech practice materials. Often the speaker must say figurative expressions "as a whole" or they lose their meaning and impact. And, the tone of some figurative expressions may need to be just right and the situational circumstance must be appropriate. Figurative expressions, particularly proverbs and adages, can sound peculiar and out of place when spoken "out of the blue," even to people who know them well and use them.

How can figurative expressions be used in therapy and with what populations?

DISORDER-SPECIFIC APPLICATIONS

Apraxia of Speech and Dysarthria

For people with apraxia of speech and/or dysarthria, figurative expressions may be useful material for addressing prosodic elements of timing/rhythm/melody, to practice a syllable-by-syllable style of speech production to maximize intelligibility, to modify speaking rate, and to address optimal loudness or to refine articulatory precision. Figurative expressions may be most useful for people with milder motor speech disorders. If language and/or other cognitive functions are impaired, as is the case most of the time with apraxia of speech and at least some of the time with dysarthria, figurative expressions may be too challenging. Yet, all things considered, as stimuli in language and cognitive rehabilitation, figurative expressions may help selected clients progress towards longer and more linguistically complex utterances, as well as to express subtle meanings.

Voice Disorders

For people with hyperfunctional voice disorders who have achieved approximated or target voice production in shorter and simpler stimuli, figurative expressions may present opportunities to practice "best possible" voice production with the affected manner and the nuances associated with saying proverbs and idioms in real-life conversations. This practice material may go well with that presented in Dialogues (Chapter 8).

Fluency

For people who stutter, figurative expressions provide many familiar comments of everyday conversations for practice of fluent speech to initiate, respond, and to build confidence.

Laryngectomy

For people who have had a total laryngectomy who use an artificial larynx device, a tracheoesophageal voice prosthesis, or use esophageal voice, and for those who have had other laryngeal surgeries, figurative expressions may be useful for practicing optimal breathing-phrasing, timing and pacing, best voice quality possible, pitch and loudness variations, and precise articulation and oral openness when speaking.

Glossectomy and Other Surgeries and Treatments for Head and Neck Cancer

For people who have had partial or total glossectomy, other head and neck surgeries, and/or chemoradiation treatments for head and neck cancer that compromise articulatory precision, figurative expressions may be used to practice compensatory articulatory gestures, to practice speaking at a slower rate and use optimal breathing-phrasing, and to experiment with pitch and prosodic variations to enhance intelligibility.

Social or Regional Dialect Modification

For people with a particular social or regional dialect variation of American English, figurative expressions may be practical material for practice of many aspects of mainstream American English. Targets for practice may include typical intonational-prosodic patterns of various sentence types, production of specific speech sounds in American English that are habitually omitted or substituted, production of all syllables in polysyllabic words, and conventional stress patterns in polysyllabic words. Figurative expressions provide opportunity for a speaker to practice the customary grammatical structure, the manner, and the speech sounds of mainstream American English.

Foreign Accent Reduction and American English as a Second Language

For people wishing to reduce their foreign accent, and for those learning American English as a second language, figurative expressions are an important component of everyday conversations in American English, yet they can be a common source of confusion. Their literal meaning is usually unrelated to the immediate circumstances of a conversation. The figurative expressions here provide material to practice a slower speaking rate to maximize intelligibility, to practice customary stress and prosodic patterns in polysyllabic words and sentences, and to learn appropriate use, tone, and other pragmatic aspects of these and other expressions that are frequently used in mainstream American English.

EXAMPLES OF GOAL AREAS AND TARGET SKILLS THAT CAN BE ADDRESSED BY FIGURATIVE EXPRESSION

Goal Areas	Target Skills
Articulation/Phonology	• specific phonemes in various word positions • consonant clusters and sound blending • polysyllabic words • overall intelligibility
Rate	• reduced speaking rate; temporal adjustments to vowels and certain consonants to increase intelligibility • increased speaking rate
Prosody	• general intonational-prosodic patterns of statements, questions and exclamations • affected style and prosody for humor, sarcasm, inference, etc. • fluency and smoothness • breath control; manner of breathing • phrasing • syllable-by-syllable production of phrases and polysyllabic words • conventional stress patterns of polysyllabic words • naturalness

Fluency	• using a prolonged-speech technique to produce specific sounds, words, and sentences • rate adjustments to preserve fluency • naturalness in prosody, timing and cadence
Voice	• increased loudness • decreased loudness • best possible voice (free of hoarseness, breathiness, and roughness with appropriate pitch and loudness) • breath support; manner of breathing • phrasing
Conversational Skills	• appropriateness • when, where, and how figurative expressions are used in conversation • conversational turn-taking; speaker-listener roles; elements of timing, tone, and style of delivery that influence meaning • initiating • responding • commenting; interjecting • quantity of discourse; abbreviating or elaborating
Social or Regional Dialect Modification	• articulation of specific speech sounds that are habitually substituted, distorted, or omitted • inclusion of all syllables of words • customary intonational-prosodic patterns of mainstream American English
Foreign Accent Reduction and American English as a Second Language	• intonational-prosodic patterns of mainstream American English • how intonation-prosody can affect the meaning of words or the entire expression • slower speaking rate to maximize intelligibility • articulation of specific speech sounds that are habitually substituted, distorted, or omitted

SUGGESTIONS FOR USING AND MODIFYING THE MATERIAL IN FIGURATIVE EXPRESSIONS

- Use highlighting, underlining, arrows, slashes, and other diacritical markings to indicate the presence of specific speech sounds, to emphasize them, to indicate pauses, alteration in rate, prolongation, change in loudness, pitch-prosodic variation, and so forth.
- Address one speech goal during one practice session, such as phrasing, then change the goal, such as to "naturalness" and placing the figurative expression into a context, during a subsequent practice of the same expressions.
- Self-monitoring and self-critique are basic to improving speech and language skills. Make audio- or video-recordings of the client producing figurative expressions. Afterward, the clinician and client play the recordings to analyze and discuss the speech performance.
- Extend or expand the task. Discuss figurative expressions with the client. Ask him or her to think of possible antecedents or follow-up comments to the expressions, for example, "Have you ever said this or something like it? "What was the situation?" or "When would you say this?" Providing a context for a particular expression may help some clients understand it better and practice it more readily. For example, the clinician might say, "When I saw the sticker price on the new car . . . ," and the client responds with the idiom, "It sent my head spinning."
- People usually make comments like those in Figurative Expressions at a fairly rapid speaking rate. Sometimes when they are spoken at a rate that is slower than customary, or when a contraction is changed to its two-word form, the cadence of the expression changes so much that the meaning is lost, the expression sounds odd, or it doesn't even sound familiar. Figurative expressions may be particularly helpful for those trying to increase their rate and to use a more natural-sounding prosody while maintaining articulatory accuracy.
- Delete or modify speech practice material that distract the client from the goals of therapy.
- Individual clients, their families, and residents of particular social groups or geographic areas have their own versions of these and other figurative expressions and sayings. Consider using the "Practice Your Own Figurative Expressions" form at the end of this chapter to practice figurative expressions familiar to the client that pertain to his or her communication style and community.

PRACTICE MATERIAL FOR FIGURATIVE EXPRESSIONS

1. Beats me
2. Dream on
3. Cool it!
4. Way to go
5. I smell a rat
6. Go fly a kite
7. Give me five
8. Holy cow!
9. Sleep on it
10. Shake a leg
11. I'm all ears
12. Get my drift?
13. Let's face it . . .
14. Heaven forbid
15. Rise and shine
16. In a nutshell . . .
17. I ate like a pig
18. You set me up
19. I'm wiped out
20. Just my luck
21. Twist my arm
22. Run for cover
23. Smarty pants!
24. He's long gone
25. So far, so good
26. You're kidding
27. He bit the dust
28. Down the hatch
29. Slowly but surely
30. Hold your horses
31. Go with the flow
32. He was framed
33. I'm tickled pink
34. Catch you later
35. What's going on?
36. I'm losing steam
37. Bite your tongue
38. To say the least
39. It's Greek to me
40. Butter fingers
41. I almost lost it
42. Connect the dots
43. He got cold feet
44. First things first
45. Get the lead out
46. He's out of touch
47. Let's call it a day
48. It's as easy as pie
49. Hold your tongue
50. That rings a bell
51. Don't make waves
52. This is no picnic
53. I'm in hot water
54. That cracks me up
55. Saved by the bell
56. Put your foot down
57. What's the point?
58. She stood me up
59. Give him a hand
60. It's a no-brainer
61. Enough is enough
62. What an air head
63. Stop bugging me
64. It's a piece of cake
65. She stole the show
66. I was so out of it

67. What a tightwad
68. That hit a nerve
69. Go the extra mile
70. Not by a long shot
71. Don't rock the boat
72. I'm a bit on edge
73. Now you're talking
74. Seeing is believing
75. It was a close call
76. Take your best shot
77. Keep your chin up
78. Age before beauty
79. That's the last straw
80. I'm as fit as a fiddle
81. This is a nightmare
82. The rest is history
83. He bought the farm
84. Shop till you drop
85. It was a false alarm
86. Eat your heart out
87. That takes the cake
88. Make up your mind
89. That ship has sailed
90. Let's hit the hay
91. Take the high road
92. Keep your shirt on!
93. Head for the hills
94. My gut feeling is . . .
95. They took up the cry
96. He's soft in the head
97. He bought the farm
98. I'm in over my head
99. He's the head honcho
100. Pull yourself together
101. This is for the birds
102. I'm at my wits' end
103. He's as cold as ice
104. Seeing is believing
105. All eyes are on her
106. I'm fed up with this
107. They flew the coop
108. He's off his rocker
109. You hit the jackpot
110. Easier said than done
111. I'm drawing a blank
112. He has a screw loose
113. Don't jump the gun
114. The tide has turned
115. Run that by me again
116. I'm fed up with this
117. He's in over his head
118. Look before you leap
119. For crying out loud!
120. He dug his own grave
121. That's the final straw
122. Oh, for heaven's sake
123. He's on his last legs
124. Then, to top it all off . . .
125. It rolls off the tongue
126. He's a tough cookie
127. Get off your high horse
128. I'll stand behind you
129. You're in good hands
130. Was that over the top?
131. Cat got your tongue?
132. He's so wishy-washy
133. It's like herding cats
134. You're full of hot air
135. I get a kick out of that
136. There's a ray of hope

137. It's like riding a bike
138. He's changed his tune
139. Keep a stiff upper lip
140. Don't be a sore loser
141. It was an eye-opener
142. The more, the merrier
143. He's lost his marbles
144. I've had it up to here
145. That was a low blow
146. She's a goody-two-shoes
147. Expect the unexpected
148. I'm on pins and needles
149. That's a sore subject
150. Then, from out of the blue . . .
151. You're in for a treat
152. It's too little, too late
153. He's a real wet blanket
154. We're down to the wire
155. I was out like a light
156. He's a real push-over
157. The sooner, the better
158. We're in the same boat
159. I can't believe my eyes
160. Practice makes perfect
161. Open mouth, insert foot
162. I get a kick out of that
163. I'll hold down the fort
164. If the shoe fits, wear it
165. Something smells fishy
166. He sure is long winded
167. She's no spring chicken
168. You're talking in circles
169. Better late than never
170. He's off in la-la land
171. That's the way it goes
172. If that doesn't beat all!
173. He kicked the bucket
174. That was the last straw
175. It's off the beaten path
176. Like a moth to a flame
177. Jump in with both feet
178. He doesn't have the guts
179. Don't get your hopes up
180. Mind your own business
181. It's as flat as a pancake
182. My life is an open book
183. He's flip-flopping again
184. Out of sight, out of mind
185. Read between the lines
186. He's living on the edge
187. Don't muddy the water
188. You dodged that bullet
189. That's pretty far fetched
190. It was bound to happen
191. Thou protests too much
192. What a blabbermouth!
193. Do as I say, not as I do
194. I was left holding the bag
195. You face an uphill battle
196. Keep your eyes peeled
197. Variety is the spice of life
198. It's an open and shut case
199. Don't try to butter me up
200. I'm just pulling your leg
201. That's a thing of the past
202. It's nothing to sneeze at
203. What do you have to lose?
204. Use a little elbow grease
205. She had me over a barrel
206. It's time to bite the bullet

207. He let the cat out of the bag
208. It went from bad to worse
209. When the dust settles . . .
210. There's just no end to it
211. It was a rude awakening
212. That's highway robbery!
213. Now I can breathe easier
214. Get your ducks in a row
215. That drives me up the wall
216. He likes to stir things up
217. Are you out of your mind?
218. I'm at the end of my rope
219. Batten down the hatches!
220. I can't put my finger on it
221. Don't worry, I don't bite
222. We have paid a high price
223. The ball is in your court
224. Will wonders never cease
225. You're headed for trouble
226. He's as busy as a beaver
227. I had to pull a few strings
228. What a bunch of babies!
229. Straighten up and fly right
230. He's as happy as a clam
231. Put your best foot forward
232. Throw caution to the wind
233. You're setting yourself up
234. I'm going to tan your hide
235. He's into it up to his elbows
236. Now I've seen everything
237. It rubs me the wrong way
238. He's a little full of himself
239. I got off on the wrong foot
240. He's as nutty as a fruitcake
241. You hit the nail on the head
242. I put myself out on a limb
243. He's gone off the deep end
244. I'll get to the bottom of this
245. He just doesn't measure up
246. I passed with flying colors
247. Stop pussy-footing around
248. He's a ticking time bomb
249. You're skating on thin ice
250. What am I? Chopped liver?
251. It was a walk in the park
252. Look what the cat dragged in
253. We're back to square one
254. Don't keep it all bottled up
255. He's going to hit the roof
256. We're getting nowhere fast
257. The road ahead looks good
258. You're a sight for sore eyes
259. She's had a colorful career
260. I got roped into it somehow
261. Honesty is the best policy
262. They had a change of heart
263. You're beating a dead horse
264. It cost me an arm and a leg
265. Are you a man or a mouse?
266. There are bigger fish to fry
267. I can't put my finger on it
268. Keep up your end of the deal
269. That's water under the bridge
270. I've been under the weather
271. They're like two peas in a pod
272. He's a fair weather friend
273. It's a pretty bleak picture
274. She put him in his place
275. Those are a dime a dozen
276. The devil is in the details

277. You get what you pay for
278. It's time to bite the bullet
279. His face was a red as a beet
280. You drive a hard bargain
281. Lay your cards on the table
282. You can't please everyone
283. Stop beating around the bush
284. He's there at her beck and call
285. All options are on the table
286. He had a complete meltdown
287. I fought it tooth and nail
288. A watched pot never boils
289. He's still calling the shots
290. Let me put in my two cents
291. He took it hook, line, and sinker
292. I won't take this lying down
293. Don't cry over spilled milk
294. He's all talk and no action
295. That threw me for a loop
296. It's not worth a hill of beans
297. They're shooting the breeze
298. Now you're on the right track
299. It's a heart-breaking situation
300. This is a recipe for disaster
301. I'm just not cut out for this
302. I got raked over the coals
303. It's like stepping back in time
304. If he plays his cards right . . .
305. That's the last thing we need
306. He's showing his true colors
307. I have to see it to believe it
308. Now he's changing his tune
309. It stopped him in his tracks
310. Let's put our heads together
311. He's living on borrowed time
312. Laughter is the best medicine
313. It will knock your socks off
314. I'm turning over a new leaf
315. That's easier said than done
316. You are taking me for granted
317. The handwriting is on the wall
318. It was a real slap in the face
319. We're not out of the woods yet
320. Finders keepers, losers weepers
321. He's always dragging his feet
322. That was too close for comfort
323. How do you like them apples?
324. I don't have the stomach for it
325. He'll end up with egg on his face
326. They're trying to make ends meet
327. You win some, you lose some
328. This is the beginning of the end
329. She gave him the cold shoulder
330. He's afraid of his own shadow
331. It's available around the clock
332. You can't hold a candle to him
333. Let's get the show on the road
334. There's no time like the present
335. No good deed goes unpunished
336. This isn't rocket science
337. You're barking up the wrong tree
338. That happens once in a blue moon
339. Victory is just around the corner
340. He must be turning in his grave
341. Don't shoot yourself in the foot
342. There's a problem at every turn
343. That's only part of the picture
344. I've had it up to here with you
345. The moment of truth is at hand
346. You'll be the death of me yet

347. Don't get all bent out of shape
348. I got more than I bargained for
349. Let's get down to the nitty-gritty
350. That's a real pain in the neck
351. He has a surprise up his sleeve
352. Every cloud has a silver lining
353. Get out while the getting is good
354. I can't make heads or tails of it
355. You are your own worst enemy
356. He can't easily be pigeonholed
357. Birds of a feather flock together
358. It's just a stone's throw away
359. His bark is worse than his bite
360. He doesn't have a leg to stand on
361. And then, from out of nowhere . . .
362. Nothing can save this train wreck
363. I can't seem to make ends meet
364. Now I can breathe a little easier
365. That's taking things a little too far
366. Beggars can't be choosers
367. Actions speak louder than words
368. Now the shoe is on the other foot
369. They pulled the plug on that plan
370. Once I get my foot in the door . . .
371. He's her knight in shining armor
372. I'm the low man on the totem pole
373. His talk is a lot of empty rhetoric
374. Don't get your nose out of joint
375. It's an accident waiting to happen
376. He ate like there's no tomorrow
377. We're waiting with bated breath
378. It was a problem from the get go
379. That's just the tip of the iceberg
380. He's a force to be reckoned with
381. Nothing ventured, nothing gained
382. From now on it's smooth sailing
383. It's enough to make your head spin
384. Well, knock me over with a feather
385. Don't put all your eggs in one basket
386. He can't see the forest from the trees
387. I just threw my hands up in the air
388. We made it by the skin of our teeth
389. You're barking up the wrong tree
390. He'll hit the roof when he finds out
391. I'm between a rock and a hard place
392. Six of one, half a dozen of the other
393. Don't let him walk all over you
394. I didn't want to ruffle any feathers
395. He's the black sheep of the family
396. That was a hair-raising experience
397. It was an eye-opening experience
398. I couldn't get a word in edgewise
399. He bit off more than he can chew
400. I'm back in the thick of things
401. The squeaky wheel gets the grease
402. He sat there like a bump on a log
403. Don't change horses in mid-stream
404. He keeps breathing down my neck
405. It's just what the doctor ordered
406. Put your money where your mouth is
407. It's like fingernails on a chalkboard
408. He's burning the candle at both ends
409. This hurts me more than it hurts you
410. It will nickel and dime you to death
411. I've tried everything under the sun
412. You can't sweep that under the rug
413. You've got to play your cards right
414. I'll give you the benefit of the doubt
415. Now he's on the straight and narrow
416. And then wham! Right in the kisser!

417. Where there's a will there's a way
418. He's a little wet behind the ears
419. He's got both feet on the ground
420. That's the way the cookie crumbles
421. When in Rome, do as the Romans do
422. Now he's throwing his weight around
423. Well, it's back to the drawing board
424. This is cruel and unusual punishment
425. It was bound to happen sooner or later
426. They've buried their heads in the sand
427. He's slower than molasses in January
428. Out of the frying pan and into the fire
429. It's a sad commentary on our society
430. Everything is gloom and doom with you
431. I don't want to step on anyone's toes
432. They had a big shake-up at the office
433. We got started off on the wrong foot
434. Give him an inch and he'll take a mile
435. You're putting the cart before the horse
436. I wouldn't touch it with a 10-foot pole
437. Things have taken a turn for the worse
438. It's got everything but the kitchen sink
439. You scratch my back, I'll scratch yours
440. He bought it lock, stock, and barrel
441. He's been around the block a few times
442. Like trying to find a needle in a haystack
443. I'm not playing second fiddle to anyone
444. Hope for the best, prepare for the worst
445. He's not the brightest bulb on the tree
446. There must be something in the water
447. He's not the sharpest knife in the drawer
448. You still haven't gotten the big picture
449. The bigger they are the harder they fall
450. What kind of half-baked excuse is that?
451. I'll spring it on him at the right moment
452. The news wasn't exactly earth shattering
453. He would give you the shirt off his back
454. Don't try to pull a fast one on me, Mister
455. You took the words right out of my mouth
456. We can no longer sit back biting our nails
457. Off the top of your head, what do you think?
458. I'm tired of always jumping through hoops
459. You could do that until the cows come home
460. There goes that idea right out the window
461. You can't put a square peg in a round hole
462. I'll knock you from here to next Tuesday
463. We'll cross that bridge when we come to it.
464. He pulled the rug right out from under me
465. What's the matter? Ants in your pants?
466. Don't think I don't know what you're up to
467. You're making a mountain out of a molehill
468. Don't give me that holier-than-thou attitude
469. You made your bed, now you can sleep in it
470. All work and no play makes Jack a dull boy

471. A bird in the hand is worth two in the bush
472. The show brought down the house
473. That kid will eat you out of house and home
474. This town ain't big enough for the two of us
475. He couldn't find his way out of a paper bag
476. I'm washing my hands of this entire situation
477. He's going around with a chip on his shoulder
478. There's something fishy going on around here
479. When the going gets tough, the tough get going
480. He'll be picking up the pieces for years to come
481. Don't count your chickens before they're hatched
482. He was parading around like he owned the place
483. Finally, I can see the light at the end of the tunnel
484. They're always trying to keep up with the Joneses
485. I bend over backward for you and this is what I get?
486. This is like rearranging the deck chairs on the Titanic
487. Other than that, Mrs. Lincoln, how did you like the play?
488. He was running around like a chicken with its head cut off
489. You can lead a horse to water but you can't make him drink.

LIMERICKS

A Tutor who tooted the flute
Tried to teach two young tooters to toot
Said the two to the Tutor,
"Is it harder to toot, or
To tutor two tooters to toot?"
by Carolyn Wells, "The Tutor"

A fly and a flea in a flue
Were imprisoned, so what could they do?
Said the fly, "Let us flee!"
"Let us fly! Said the flea,
So they flew through a flaw in the flue.
Anonymous

A bottle of perfume that Willie sent
Was highly displeasing to Millicent.
Her thanks were so cold
That they quarreled, I'm told
Through that silly scent Willie sent Millicent.
Anonymous

She frowned and called him Mr.
Because in sport he kr.
And so in spite
That very nite
This Mr. kr. sr.
Anonymous

There was a young fellow named Hall
Who fell in the spring in the fall.
'Twould have been a sad thing
Had he died in the spring,
But he didn't—he died in the fall.
Anonymous

There was an old man of Nantucket
Who kept all his cash in a bucket
But his daughter, named Nan,
Ran away with a man,
And as for the bucket, Nantucket
Anonymous

There once was an old man of Lyme
Who married three wives at a time.
When asked, "Why a third?"
He replied, "One's absurd!
And bigamy, sir, is a crime."
Anonymous

A canner, exceedingly canny,
One morning remarked to his granny,
"A canner can can
Anything that he can,
But a canner can't can a can, can he?
Carolyn Wells, "The Canner"

There was a young man of Laconia,
Whose mother-in-law had pneumonia.
He hoped for the worst—
And after March first
They buried her 'neath a begonia.
Anonymous

There was a young lady of Bright
Whose speed was much faster than light.
She set out one day
In a relative way
And returned on the previous night.
Anonymous

I sat next to the Duchess at tea;
It was just as I feared it would be:
Her rumblings abdominal
Were truly phenomenal,
And everyone thought it was me!
Woodrow Wilson

A newspaper writer named Fling
Could make copy from most anything;
But the copy he wrote
Of a ten-dollar note
Was so good he's now in Sing-Sing
Anonymous

"PRACTICE YOUR OWN FIGURATIVE EXPRESSIONS" FORM

Make a list of figurative expressions you say or that others say in your family or community. Then practice them. Tell yourself, "When I say these, I will keep this goal in mind":

Goal: ____

____

1. ____

2. ____

3. ____

4. ____

5. ____

6. ____

7. ____

8. ____

9. ____

10. ____

7

Speaking with Exaggerated Articulatory Movements

This chapter presents practice material for speaking with increased oral openness and exaggerated articulatory movements, also referred to as "overarticulation." The intended outcome is for the client to practice more precise articulation, prolonged vowels and diphthongs, increased loudness, slower speaking rate, and increased intelligibility. The sentences contain more than the average number of vowels and diphthongs that can be produced fairly naturally with an exaggerated, more open mouth posture than others. These are /eɪ/ as in "bait," /æ/ in "bat," /ɑ/ in "pot," /aʊ/ as in "out," /aɪ/ as in "bite," /er/ in "bear," and /ɑr/ in "bark." In addition, when the client speaks with greater oral openness the clinician can better observe the client's intraoral articulatory patterns, and if necessary, guide him or her to more precise gestures. Sometimes clients will exaggerate oral openness but they do not exaggerate lingual and labial articulatory movements. These clients usually catch on to the task with additional cuing and feedback from the clinician. Also, clients may say they feel odd opening their mouth more and emphasizing articulatory placements, and that the resulting speech sounds unusual to them. There is little doubt that prosody under these conditions will be somewhat unnatural. However, the all important outcome of improved intelligibility may be achieved or approximated, and with the clinician's guidance, some of the more conspicuous speech movements may be gradually reduced without loss of intelligibility.

As with all speech practice material in this manual, the clinician determines how to use it and with whom. Practicing exaggerated articulatory movements may be only one step in a continuum of management techniques to achieve a specific goal. For some clients, exaggerated articulation may be the ultimate goal of intervention. If overarticulation causes a degree of unnaturalness that is too distracting for the client, this approach probably should be discontinued.

How can speaking with exaggerated articulatory movements be used in therapy and with what populations?

DISORDER-SPECIFIC APPLICATIONS

Apraxia of Speech and Dysarthria

For people with apraxia of speech and/or dysarthria, speaking with exaggerated articulatory movements reduces rate. Decreased rate may provide additional time for motor planning and/or programming for more precise articulation, and more time to reach targets. Also, it may facilitate processes of sensory feedback.

Laryngectomy

Laryngectomized people often must increase articulatory precision and oral openness especially when they use an artificial larynx device, and sometimes when they speak with tracheoesophageal puncture or use esophageal voice. Exaggerated articulation and more open mouth postures when speaking can dramatically improve intelligibility. For many clients it is important to introduce the concept of overarticulation early in the process of voice-speech rehabilitation.

Glossectomy and Other Head and Neck Cancer Surgeries and Treatments

People who have had head and neck cancer and who have undergone one or a combination of treatments including surgery, radiation therapy, and chemotherapy, often suffer from loss of tissue or limited jaw, lip, and tongue movement that cause omissions and distortions of speech sounds and aberrant, hard-to-understand speech. Other speech and swallowing problems may show up months and years after surgical and medical treatments, even in the absence of recurrent or new disease. Many of these individuals improve their intelligibility when they exaggerate articulatory movements. Yet, this is not always true. When the palate or tongue is surgically altered and/or tongue movement is significantly impaired, some people may be more intelligible when they speak with reduced or restricted jaw openness. In any case, encourage clients to move their tongue, lips, and jaw while speaking rather than their head.

Foreign Accent Reduction and American English as a Second Language

People with a foreign accent and those learning American English as a second language often require specific instruction on how to articulate certain speech sounds of American English and how to make them precisely. When these clients speak with exaggerated articulation the clinician can more readily examine their speech movements, help correct their error patterns and idiosyncrasies, and help guide them to their best production of American English.

EXAMPLES OF GOAL AREAS AND TARGET SKILLS THAT CAN BE ADDRESSED BY SPEAKING WITH EXAGGERATED ARTICULATORY MOVEMENTS

Goal Areas	Target Skills
Articulation/Phonology	• additional time for motor planning and/or programming • facilitating sensory feedback • precise kinematics for specific phonemes in various word positions • consonant clusters and sound blending • intelligibility
Rate	• reducing speaking rate • intelligibility
Prosody	• exaggeration of intonation-melody of verbal expression • conventional intonation-stress patterns of polysyllabic words and various sentence types
Voice	• increased loudness • pitch variation • best possible voice (free of hoarseness, breathiness, roughness with appropriate pitch and loudness)
Conversational Skills	• increased intelligibility • more willing, engaged and comfortable communication partners when the client's speech is more intelligible
Social or Regional Dialect Modification	• articulation of specific phonemes that are habitually omitted, substituted, or distorted • inclusion of all syllables of words • intonation-prosodic patterns of mainstream American English
Foreign Accent Reduction and English as a Second Language	• slower speaking rate • prosodic-intonational patterns of statements, questions, and exclamations of American English • stress patterns of polysyllabic words • inclusion of all syllables of words • intelligibility • articulation of specific phonemes that are habitually substituted, omitted, or distorted

SUGGESTIONS FOR USING AND MODIFYING THE MATERIAL IN SPEAKING WITH EXAGGERATED ARTICULATORY MOVEMENTS

- Use highlighting, underlining, arrows, slashes, and other diacritical markings to indicate where to exaggerate oral openness, to indicate the presence of specific speech sounds, to emphasize them, to indicate pauses, alteration in rate, prolongation of vowels, change in loudness, pitch-prosodic variation, and so forth.
- Substitute vocabulary to increase or decrease the occurrence of specific speech sounds or occurrence of polysyllabic words as needed for a particular client.
- Ask the client to read or say the sentences several times and to use a different prosody each time. Model various prosodic patterns as necessary. Add or substitute words or make other alterations to personalize or to enhance the impact of the exercise.
- Speakers may make additional and unnecessary facial and head movements when they emphasize and exaggerate speech movements. Video recordings or practice in front of a mirror with the clinician's guidance early in the exercise will help the client recognize and eliminate non-speech movements.
- Appearing and sounding natural and normal are obvious and desired endpoints to speech and language therapy. Clinicians may be concerned that when some clients practice speaking with exaggerated articulatory movements, to the point of appearing conspicuous, the exaggerated movements may carry over to the client's everyday manner of speaking. This rarely, if ever, occurs. If a client exhibits a particularly undesirable speech behavior or pattern, the clinician's model and cues can help shape unusual movements into more acceptable behavior soon after it begins.
- Self-monitoring and self-critique are basic to improving speech skills. A goal is for the client to recognize his speech errors, become aware of his approximations to speech targets, and realize when he has reached target performance. Again, the clinician may audio- or video-record the client reading or repeating the stimuli, then review the recordings with the client to analyze the speech performance. With the emphasis on exaggerated speech movements, video recordings may provide particularly revealing and instructive feedback.
- Some clients rarely hear positive comments about their speech from family members. Positive feedback from family and friends can be powerful reinforcement for the person who usually hears negative questions and comments about his speech, such as, "What did you say?" "Huh?" "I don't get it" or "Say it louder." With the client's permission, invite his significant others into the therapy session at critical moments when the client is doing particularly well, and ask them to comment on the improved speech performance. This is uplifting for everyone and may help the client realize how exaggerated articulatory movements can truly improve speech.
- To vary this material, the speech-language pathologist and client may think of antecedents or follow-up comments to the sentences using the same exaggerated articulatory style. With the exception of some question marks and exclamation marks, punctuation at the ends of the sentences has been omitted to promote longer utter-

ances or additional comments. Consider presenting the sentences in the question-answer format of Contrastive Stress Drills (Chapter 9). For a silly-and-strange version of these stimuli, link two of the shorter sentences with "and," "or," "but," or "and, by the way." Example: "Fat chance . . . and, by the way . . . I look great!" All variations of the stimuli and the task are encouraged as long as they complement the goals of therapy.

- For additional and longer material for practicing exaggerated articulatory movements, consider oral reading of simple poems or the lyrics of selected songs that may be fairly naturally recited with exaggerated articulatory movements, such as "Let It Be," "California Dreamin," and "Yellow Submarine."
- Whatever the purpose for selecting this material for use in therapy, part of the clinician's role is to describe to the client and demonstrate what he or she can do to improve his speech. Consider demonstrating the target speech behavior frequently during therapy sessions until these models can be faded.
- Delete or change any stimuli that distract the client from the intended therapy goals.
- Based on the clinician's experience, the etiology and type of a client's speech disorder, and the evidence available in the speech-language pathology literature, it may be appropriate to recommend specific oral/nonverbal movements or exercises to complement the speech practice material presented here. For example, people who have had medical treatments for head and neck cancer may benefit from exercises to increase the speed and/or range of motion of the tongue, lips, and jaw.
- Consider using the form, "Practice Speaking with Exaggerated Movements" at the end of this chapter to individualize material for a client to practice outside the therapy session.

PRACTICE MATERIAL FOR SPEAKING WITH EXAGGERATED ARTICULATORY MOVEMENTS

1. Hi
2. Bye
3. Ouch!
4. Why not?
5. No way!
6. I'm ahead
7. Ship ahoy!
8. I'll be back
9. Fat chance
10. I look great
11. That's awful
12. Go fly a kite
13. How are you?
14. Call the cops
15. Shout out loud
16. I'll eat my hat
17. What a shock!
18. Get out of here
19. Out damn spot!
20. I'm fine, thanks
21. Don't talk back
22. Out of my way!
23. What's up, Doc?
24. Up, up, and away
25. I ate a pile of crab
26. My how time flies!
27. I can't walk that far
28. Is there time for pie?
29. For crying out loud!
30. That's a lot of typing
31. How now brown cow?
32. Where are the clouds?
33. Take a big bite of cake
34. I can't tuck in my coat
35. That lady has a fine tan
36. We all had a great time
37. Hey, buddy, got a dime?
38. I gave all the cash I had
39. What time does it chime?
40. Lights! Camera! Action!
41. My coffee is not at all hot
42. They ran down to the car
43. I stayed up late that night
44. Put another log on the fire
45. That guy botched the job
46. Why that guy and not me?
47. We will dine in a fine café
48. I saw "Some Like It Hot"
49. Are you out of your mind?
50. He sawed logs all night long
51. And don't come back, Jack
52. My mail was late again today
53. Mom's wild rice tastes great
54. I rode my bike up Pike's Peak
55. I don't play the blame game
56. That's tall talk for a shy guy
57. Oh, great! More hate mail
58. Our band played all night long
59. I had a rash all over my back
60. She vowed to have my hide
61. If I were king of the forest . . .
62. Plant plenty of carrots and peas
63. I hate that loud alarm clock
64. How long can five dollars last?

65. I have not yet begun to fight
66. That backpack can hold a lot
67. Attention Wal-Mart shoppers
68. Oh, waiter. Where is my pie?
69. My black eye aches like crazy
70. The tree was five feet too high
71. A giant gnat bit me on the back
72. My hand got caught in the gate
73. We like to bike around the lake
74. I'm ready for a hot cup of coffee
75. Our band jammed all night long
76. They were outraged by the sight
77. I nagged my boss and I got fired
78. Hail knocked down half of the crop
79. Get that black cat out of my chair
80. Isn't this a revolting development!
81. My team doesn't have much steam
82. I vow I won't take this lying down
83. The only thing to fear is fear itself
84. Would you like to swing on a star?
85. How about some pie and ice cream?
86. The scent of pine was mighty strong
87. My Mom's hamburger hash is awful
88. I don't want to set the world on fire
89. My mail got sent to the wrong house
90. My dog tore down the shower curtain
91. I finally found that awful white bow tie
92. Where in the world did that come from?
93. My back yard is a lake after all that rain
94. Up, up, and away in my beautiful balloon
95. I want apple pie with ice cream piled high
96. The rain in Spain stays mainly on the plain
97. I've got to lie down on the couch for a while
98. He was exhausted after he walked up that trail
99. Icy sidewalks caused him to fall flat on his back
100. My watchdog, Fido, yawned as the robber ran off
101. I scream, you scream, we all scream for ice cream
102. Jack, talk with your mouth open, but eat with it closed
103. Remember the cow that ate all my flowers down to the ground? Well, have another steak!
104. "You have the right to remain silent. Anything you say can and will be used against you in a court of law. You have the right to have an attorney present during questioning. If you cannot afford an attorney, one will be appointed."
105. "Now, Dasher! Now, Dancer! Now, Prancer and Vixen! On Comet, On Cupid, On Donner and Blitzen! To the top of the porch! To the top of the wall! Now dash away! Dash away! Dash away all!"

"PRACTICE SPEAKING WITH EXAGGERATED MOVEMENTS" FORM

Write words, phrases or sentences you say frequently. Examples: "See you later!" "Are you serious?" "What's for dinner?" Then practice saying these with exaggerated speech movements.

Goal: ______________________________

____

1. ______________________________

2. ______________________________

3. ______________________________

4. ______________________________

5. ______________________________

6. ______________________________

7. ______________________________

8. ______________________________

9. ______________________________

10. ______________________________

8

Dialogues

These dialogues are scripted conversations for two people. Scripted conversations capture the back-and-forth character of natural conversations and provide a framework for presenting specific stimuli for speech practice. Each dialogue is made up of everyday vocabulary and short sentences with each speaker taking short turns. Occasionally, some of the sentences and speaking turns are longer and the vocabulary is not as common. Most of the dialogues contain stereotyped characters, familiar expressions, figurative language, and quotations. Humor is an obvious element of the dialogues.

Like all material in this manual, the dialogues are meant to be customized by the speech-language pathologist based on a client's speech-language-communication diagnosis, goal areas, and speech targets, and the client's abilities, background, and preferences. To write original dialogues, refer to the "Write and Practice Your Own Dialogues" form at the end of this chapter.

How can dialogues be used in therapy and with what populations?

DISORDER-SPECIFIC APPLICATIONS

Apraxia of Speech and Dysarthria

People with apraxia of speech or dysarthria often have associated aphasic language impairment and linguistically based speech errors. Consider using dialogues for a client with a mild motor speech disorder to practice self-correction of sound errors, speaking slower or faster, or to prolong certain speech sounds, to address habitually misarticulated words, to practice a more natural cadence, or to modify breathing or phrasing. Dialogues may be useful material for practicing articulatory precision, improved rate, loudness, and timing/rhythm/melody. There are many speech, language, and communication goals that can be addressed with scripted conversations as long as the client's speech, language and/or cognitive impairment is mild-to-mild/moderate, and he or she can read aloud.

Non-Aphasic Cognitive Impairment

For people with non-aphasic cognitive impairment such as that associated with traumatic brain injury, and whether or not a motor speech disorder is present, dialogues may be helpful for addressing various pragmatic aspects of language, such as speaker and listener roles, understanding subtleties of language, tone of voice, style that changes with varying communicative situations, and conversational etiquette. Dialogues may also be used to address non-speech related therapy goals such as attention, memory, problem solving, and thinking of alternatives.

Laryngectomy

For people who have had a total laryngectomy who use an artificial larynx device, a tracheo-esophageal voice prosthesis, or esophageal voice, and for those who have had other laryngeal surgeries, the material in this section may be helpful for practicing improved coordination of breathing-phrasing, timing and pacing, emphasis and stress, as well as for addressing loudness and voice quality that affect intelligibility and overall communicative effectiveness.

Glossectomy and Other Head and Neck Cancer Surgeries and Treatments

For people who have had partial or total glossectomy, other head and neck surgeries, and/or chemoradiation treatments for head and neck cancer that compromise articulatory precision, this material may be used to explore and practice compensatory articulatory gestures, to practice speaking at a reduced rate, and to experiment with pitch and prosodic variations to enhance intelligibility.

Fluency

For people who stutter, dialogues may be helpful for practicing specific fluency techniques in simulated conversation, to address dysfluencies on specific sounds or words, and to achieve more natural timing and prosody. Consider writing original dialogues that incorporate easy-to-difficult speaking situations, speech sounds, and vocabulary.

Social or Regional Dialect Modification

For people with a social or regional dialect variation of American English, dialogues may be particularly helpful for practicing many aspects of mainstream American English. Targets for practice may include typical intonational-prosodic patterns of various sentence types, production of specific speech sounds that are habitually deleted or substituted, production of all syllables in polysyllabic words when some are usually deleted, and stress patterns in polysyllabic words.

Foreign Accent and American English as a Second Language

For people wishing to reduce their foreign accent and for those learning American English as a second language, dialogues provide rich material to practice articulation of specific sounds, to practice a slower speaking rate to maximize intelligibility, and to practice customary stress and prosodic patterns in polysyllabic words and in phrases. In addition, dialogues provide opportunity for actual use of American English—use of tone and timing to influence meaning, use of slang and abbreviated utterances, figurative language, colloquial expressions, and the innumerable pragmatic aspects of speech and language in communication.

EXAMPLES OF GOAL AREAS AND TARGET SKILLS THAT CAN BE ADDRESSED BY DIALOGUES

Goal Areas	Target Skills
Articulation/Phonology	• specific phonemes in all word positions • consonant clusters and sound blending • polysyllabic words • mainstream American English • overall intelligibility
Rate	• reduced speaking rate • increased speaking rate
Prosody	• customary intonational-prosodic patterns of statements, questions, and exclamations • affected style and prosody for humor, sarcasm, etc. • conversational rhythm and timing of mainstream American English • conventional stress patterns of polysyllabic words • fluency and smoothness • manner of breathing; breath control • phrasing • naturalness
Fluency	• using a prolonged-speech technique for specific sounds, words, and phrases in simulated conversation • practicing nonavoidance of specific speech sounds, words, conversational circumstances
Voice	• best possible voice (free of hoarseness, breathiness, roughness and with appropriate pitch and loudness) • increased loudness • reduced loudness • vary loudness-intonation with the conversational circumstance • breath support; manner of breathing • phrasing

Conversational Skills	• rules of conversation—when, where, and how of speaking in various conversational circumstances • conversational turn-taking and speaker-listener roles • elements of timing that influence meaning • initiating • responding • topic maintenance • commenting; interjecting • quantity of discourse; abbreviating or elaborating • style of interaction • conversational etiquette • appropriateness • naturalness
Social or Regional Dialect Modification	• articulation of specific speech sounds of American English that are habitually omitted, substituted, or distorted • inclusion of all syllables of words • intonational-prosodic patterns of mainstream American English
Foreign Accent Reduction and American English as a Second Language	• slower speaking rate to maximize intelligibility • customary intonational-prosodic patterns of conversational mainstream American English • articulation of specific speech sounds that are habitually omitted, substituted or distorted • inclusion of all syllables of words • how changing elements of prosody can change the meaning of words or an entire phrase • use of common expressions and figurative language in American English conversation • naturalness • conversational etiquette

SUGGESTIONS FOR USING AND MODIFYING THE PRACTICE MATERIAL IN DIALOGUES

- After going through a dialogue with a client for the first time to learn what it is about, prepare for subsequent readings by indicating what target speech behaviors will be practiced. Use highlighting, underlining, arrows, slashes, and other diacritical markings to indicate the presence of specific speech sounds, to emphasize-stress them, to indicate pauses, alteration in rate, prolongation, change in loudness, pitch-prosodic variation, and so forth.
- The back and forth turn-taking of conversations is taken to an extreme in these dialogues. Most of the conversational turns are quite short, whereas, in real-life conversations, speaking, and listening roles are probably longer, and usually there is not such a strict back-and-forth cadence to the exchange. Lengthen or shorten the conversational turns of the dialogues based on the client's speech and language capabilities and needs.
- Address one of the client's speech goals, such as overall intelligibility, during one reading of a dialogue, then change the goal—such as to phrasing or naturalness—during a subsequent practice of the same dialogue.
- Substitute vocabulary to increase or decrease the occurrence of specific speech sounds or occurrence of polysyllabic words. Alter sentences to complement the client's language capabilities, communication style, and common social interactions.
- Exaggerate the characters/personalities in the dialogues using extreme styles and prosodic characteristics while maintaining the intended therapy goals and targets.
- Conversations in real life can move along very quickly, and when we read printed dialogue, our natural tendency seems to be to read it rapidly. Yet, the pathway to attaining goals in speech and language therapy often requires the client to respond in a slower, contemplative manner, to "hit" all the targets, and to self-correct errors. The clinician sets the pace in these scripted conversations. When taking a turn in the dialogues consider modeling a slower than normal speed of discourse and exaggerate the client's speech targets. Emphasize to the client that accuracy comes first, speed comes later.
- Each dialogue can be modified and used a number of times with a particular client. For example, the speech-language pathologist and client may think of possible antecedents or follow-up comments that are individualized to the client's goals. Ask the client, "If you were in this situation, what would you say?" or "If this were real life, what do you think the character would say here?" or "What will happen next?" As another example, when the client achieves the target speech behaviors during oral reading, consider paraphrasing the same conversation and "performing" it without the script. The client may need to be reminded that the goal of this activity is to maintain the target speech performance.
- These dialogues are written for two people, but they can be used effectively in group therapy settings in a variety of ways.
- Self-monitoring and self-critique are fundamental to improving speech and conversational skills. A long used and valuable therapy technique is to make audio- or video-recordings of the client participating in the dialogues, then the clinician and client review the recordings to discuss and analyze the client's speech performance.
- Speech therapy can be hard work for the client and the clinician. Most if not all of

the dialogues in this chapter are intended to be humorous, if not outright silly. Enjoy them. Skip the ones that don't work or rewrite them so they are more natural and client-specific. Some topics for consideration: a simulated conversation between the client and his employer; asking a question or responding to a question in a classroom; rehearsing a conversation with a physician, auto mechanic, or salesperson; being disciplined; asking for a pay raise; simulating a job interview; discussion about what to wear on a first date; conversation on a first date; or ordering a meal at a restaurant or fast food counter.

- A simple form to write your own client-specific dialogues appears on the last page of this chapter.

PRACTICE MATERIAL FOR DIALOGUES

Swimming

Mike's a swimmer. Jack isn't.

Jack: Hi, Mike.
Mike: Hi, Jack.
Jack: How are you doing?
Mike: I'm pretty good. How are you?
Jack: Pretty good. Boy, it sure is cold out.
Mike: I know. I hope it warms up soon.
Jack: Me, too.
Mike: Have you been in the pool yet?
Jack: Yeah. It was freezing!
Mike: That's strange. This pool is usually pretty warm.
Jack: I'm still freezing.
Mike: Huh! Swimming usually warms me up fast.
Jack: I don't swim. I float and bob.
Mike: What do you mean?
Jack: I just float around on my back, and if the water isn't too deep, I bob up and down.
Mike: You know, swimming is really good exercise. And it'll warm you up.
Jack: What about bobbing?
Mike: I don't think so.

How Many More Miles?

A man is driving with his young daughter and son. The trip feels like it is getting longer, not shorter.

Anna: Dad, are we there yet?
Dad: No, but it won't be long.
Anna: How many more miles?
Dad: One mile less than when you asked me a minute ago.
Anna: Alex, stop looking at me!
Dad: Alex, please stop looking at your sister.
Anna: He's still looking.
Dad: Come on, guys! My patience is wearing thin.
Anna: Yeah, Alex. Knock it off.
Dad: Anna, I'm talking to you, too.
Anna: Dad, I have to go to the bathroom.
Dad: You went 15 minutes ago.
Anna: I have to go again.

Dad: You'll just have to hang on a little longer.
Anna: But, I'll explode!
Dad: No, you won't.
Anna: Yes I will. Alex, stop looking at me!
Dad: I'm ready to stop the car and make you kids walk there.
Anna: Dad, it's against the law to abandon your children.
Dad: (Sigh!) How many more miles?

TV Commercial

Husband: Look. There it is again.
Wife: What?
Husband: That commercial I told you about.
Wife: What about it?
Husband: The wife and the kids are ganging up on the man.
Wife: Oh, they're just teasing him a little.
Husband: A little? They're treating him like he can't even think!
Wife: I think it's kind of cute.
Husband: No, it's more than that. Look what the wife is doing.
Wife: You're reading too much into it.
Husband: See the looks the woman and the children are giving each other? They're saying to themselves, "Dad sure is thick between the ears." What kind of message is that for kids?
Wife: Take it easy. I think you're taking it a little too seriously.
Husband: Sure. He's probably the breadwinner, but even the three-year-old knows more than he does.
Wife: It's just a commercial. Don't watch it if it bothers you so much.
Husband: You would never see a commercial where the husband and kids treat the mother like she was stupid. Women would rise up and protest. It would be off the air in no time. The company would probably go out of business.
Wife: Maybe you're right. But, don't you think it's kind of funny? I think a lot of men act that way. Not that much, of course, but a little.
Husband: Oh, I suppose so. There's no doubt that guy's a real idiot. Boy, I'm glad I'm not that way.
Wife: I suppose . . .

Sorry, Wrong Number

A hungry man dials a wrong telephone number.

Woman: Hello.
Man: Yeah, I'd like two medium pizzas with the works.
Woman: What? Sorry, but you have the wrong number.
Man: Yeah, right. I'd like them delivered as soon as . . .
Woman: I told you, you have the wrong number.

Man: Isn't this Wally's Pizza World?
Woman: No.
Man: Kris? Is that you? I didn't think you worked today.
Woman: I'm not Kris. This isn't Wally's Pizza World.
Man: Oh, come on, Kris. I need those pizzas! Extra cheese. Pronto!
Woman: Like I said, I'm not Kris. Wait a minute . . . is this you, Max?
Man: No, I'm Jim. Quit goofing around. I want those pizzas.
Woman: I've got to admit, Max, this is the wildest one you've come up with yet.
Man: This is Kris, isn't it?
Woman: No. And you don't sound like Max.
Man: That's because my name is Jim. And this isn't Wally's, is it?
Woman: No.
Man: Isn't this 234-5678?
Woman: No, but you're close.
Man: Oops! Sorry, wrong number.
Woman: That's okay. This is the weirdest call I've ever received!

If the Shoe Fits

A woman finds the perfect pair of shoes at a shoe store. But, there's a small problem.

Salesperson: Hello. May I help you?
Customer: Yes. I'd like to see these in a size 7½.
Salesperson: That's a popular size. I'm not sure . . .
Customer: I really want these shoes.
Salesperson: I'll look on the computer to see what we have.
Customer: They'll be perfect with my new outfit.
Salesperson: It looks like we only have them in 6½.
Customer: Let me see them. I think they'll fit.
Salesperson: Here, I'll measure your feet.
Customer: Don't bother. They're 7½.
Salesperson: They look more like an 8—or larger.
Customer: Just let me try the shoes you have!
Salesperson: Here they are, but there's no way you will fit into these.
Customer: Ugh! I'll keep pushing. Use a shoehorn.
Salesperson: I already am using a shoehorn.
Customer: Here, let me try.
Salesperson: You're going to damage the shoes!
Customer: I'll get them stretched at a shoe repair shop.
Salesperson: They won't stretch that much.
Customer: Are you saying I have big feet?
Salesperson: I'm saying your feet are not size 6½.
Customer: I'm saying you are rude, and I'm wearing my new shoes home.
Salesperson: Well, the customer is always right . . . I guess.

We're Not Lost!

A man and his wife are on their way to a wedding reception. He is driving and cannot find the reception hall.

Man: This looks very familiar.
Woman: You said that when we drove by here 15 minutes ago.
Man: I'm sure it's up here on the left.
Woman: Here we go again.
Man: What do you mean, "Here we go again?"
Woman: Every time we go somewhere it's the same.
Man: Oh, come on!
Woman: You are too stubborn to ask for directions.
Man: I don't need directions.
Woman: We've been lost for a half hour.
Man: We're not lost.
Woman: Oh, please.
Man: We're not lost. I know we're in the right area.
Woman: Let's stop at that service station.
Man: We don't need gas.
Woman: No, but we need directions.
Man: No, we don't.
Woman: For Pete's sake! You're acting just like my father.
Man: And you're acting exactly like my mother.
Woman: Why don't you just admit that you . . .
Man: Ah ha! There it is on the right. I told you I knew where I was going.
Woman: What do you know! And this time we're only 30 minutes late.

Complaint Department

A dissatisfied customer is returning a shirt to a department store.

Clerk: Good morning. May I help you?
Customer: You most certainly may.
Clerk: What seems to be the problem?
Customer: I bought this shirt here last week. I want my money back.
Clerk: What's wrong with it.
Customer: See for yourself.
Clerk: It looks like it has been washed.
Customer: Look a little closer. See? The seams are coming apart.
Clerk: Hmm . . . Yes, I see that.
Customer: I put it in the washer for the first time this morning and this is how it came out.
Clerk: Did you wash it according to the directions on the tag?

Customer: Of course! I like the shirt but this is simply unacceptable.
Clerk: Do you have the sales receipt?
Customer: There wasn't a reason to keep it. The shirt looked fine when I bought it.
Clerk: I'm sorry, but we don't accept returns without a sales receipt.
Customer: What? Your store brand is on the tag. And, all the sales people here know me. I want my money back!
Clerk: I'm sorry, madam, but my supervisor will have to handle this.
Customer: Who is your supervisor?
Clerk: Her name is Mrs. Dean.
Customer: Oh, not her! I'd rather talk with Mr. Taylor. He's much more understanding.
Clerk: Then, you've been here before?
Customer: Oh, yes, many times. Usually about once a week. There are just so many inferior products on the market nowadays.
Clerk: I see. Well, I'm certain Mrs. Dean will be delighted to see you. I'll get her.

Mother-in-Law

A man returns home from work and unexpectedly finds his mother-in-law.

Woman: Hello.
Man: What? Where's Deb?
Woman: Out looking for a part-time job.
Man: What for?
Woman: To supplement your salary.
Man: Huh?
Woman: To make some money. Someone has to bring home the bacon.
Man: She didn't tell me she was looking for a job.
Woman: Are you surprised?
Man: Well, sort of. When did she leave?
Woman: About three hours ago. I hear you're up to your neck in debt.
Man: Well, things could be better, but we're getting by.
Woman: It sounds pretty grim to me.
Man: That's our business!
Woman: Oh? Deb is my daughter, you know.
Man: I realize that, but . . . why are you here anyway?
Woman: I just wanted to help out in the little ways I can.
Man: Deb didn't tell me you would be here.
Woman: Maybe you should talk with her sometime instead of staying so long at the office.
Man: That's none of your business either.
Woman: Calm down. The last thing I want to do is to interfere. Far be it from me to cause a stir. By the way, have you asked your boss for a raise yet?

A Missing Sock

Man: Honey, I can't find my other sock.
Woman: Which one?
Man: My favorite. The brown one with the diamonds on the side.
Woman: That's called argyle.
Man: Okay. Where is my argyle sock?
Woman: How would I know?
Man: You did the laundry, didn't you?
Woman: Of course. I always do the laundry. And, I wash whatever is in the basket.
Man: How could only one sock get washed?
Woman: Maybe you put only one sock in the basket.
Man: Why would I do that? You must have dropped it or something.
Woman: I doubt it.
Man: Well, how can a sock disappear?
Woman: It sounds like you are accusing me of losing it.
Man: If the sock fits!
Woman: All right, my dear. I have a terrific solution to this problem.
Man: Never mind. I know where you're going with this. I don't like those socks that much! These black socks are my new favorites.

Door-to-Door Salesman

A door-to-door salesman knocks on the wrong door.

Woman: Yes?
Salesman: Good afternoon, madam. I represent the Lotsa Brushes Company. Our motto is "If it's got bristles, we've got it."
Woman: I'm not interested, thank you.
Salesman: Please don't be too hasty, madam. I carry a line of excellent products at prices that are hard to pass up.
Woman: If I needed a brush, I'd buy it at the local hardware store.
Salesman: I am local. That's why I'm here.
Woman: How long have you been in town, and why haven't I seen you before?
Salesman: I just moved here.
Woman: When?
Salesman: Yesterday.
Woman: Just as I thought, a temporary relocation, no doubt. You'll be gone soon. If I buy a brush and it falls apart, you'll be long gone.
Salesman: Oh, we guarantee all our products. You can always get an exchange. Just contact us.
Woman: Don't give me that line, buster. You fly-by-night operators are all alike. You move into a small town, sell all your products, and then you take off.
Salesman: Madame, you do me injustice!
Woman: Say, do you have a permit to sell door-to-door in this town?

Salesman: There is no such thing.
Woman: You're wrong. In this little town it's required. Show me your permit or I'll call the cops.
Salesman: That will not be necessary, madam.
Woman: Then hit the road, Jack.
Salesman: My goodness, it's 4 o'clock already! I've got to run. Good day, madam.

Fractured Quotations

A high school student is studying for a test. Her older brother isn't very helpful.

Jason: Sara, your room looks like a demolition site.
Sara: I can't do anything about it now.
Jason: When did the tornado hit?
Sara: Very funny. Now get out of here.
Jason: But Mom's in a crabby mood and she wants us to help clean the house.
Sara: Well, I have a big test on famous quotations tomorrow and I'm not ready for it.
Jason: You're in luck. I'm great at that stuff.
Sara: Lucky me.
Jason: I'm serious. How about this one, "I have a dream . . . " that you will clean your room sometime this century.
Sara: That is so lame. Out!
Jason: Or, "I only regret that I have but one . . . " bedroom to keep clean and tidy.
Sara: Jason! Be stupid someplace else. I need to study!
Jason: "Four score and seven years ago . . . " was the last time anyone could enter your room without tripping over something and nearly breaking their neck.
Sara: Go away!
Jason: I like this one, "Ask not what your . . . " brother can do for you, ask what you can do for your brother.
Sara: Do you want me to flunk my test? How am I supposed to remember the real quotes when you mess them up like that?
Jason: Just take 10 minutes and make a pathway through this mess or Mom's going to start yelling.
Sara: But, I've got to study.
Jason: Look, I can help you with the quotes later, but start cleaning up now. If Mom starts yelling at you, she'll find something to yell at me about.

Haircut

Ben: Dad, now that I have my license, can I use the car tonight?
Dad: Ben, we've talked about this already.
Ben: Yeah, but look at everything I've accomplished.
Dad: You've certainly made some nice improvements.
Ben: Yep, it's just like we bargained.

Dad: You certainly have been studying more and bringing up your grades.
Ben: Yep. Ask me anything about the religions of the world. I bet I know the answer.
Dad: Very impressive. Now there's only one more thing and you know what it is.
Ben: Yeah, but . . .
Dad: Ben, don't "yeah, but" me. You still haven't gotten your hair cut.
Ben: But, Dad, I've been thinking about that and I have something to show you. Have you looked at the pictures in my religion book?
Dad: No.
Ben: Well, look at this. Do you notice anything in particular?
Dad: Like what?
Ben: Here. These are pictures of the important people in all the religions of the world from thousands of years ago. They all had long hair! Every one! Just look!
Dad: I see.
Ben: Here's one with hair down to his shoulders.
Dad: You're right, his hair is pretty long.
Ben: This one has long hair stacked up on his head.
Dad: Uh-huh.
Ben: And this one is almost bald, but he has a long braid.
Dad: I see what you're getting at.
Ben: All right! So I can borrow the car?
Dad: Hold on a second. Have you noticed anything else about the people in these pictures?
Ben: Like what?
Dad: Look closely.
Ben: I don't see anything else.
Dad: They're all walking.
Ben: Awwww, Dad . . .

A Second Chance

David failed another history test. Now he is having a student-teacher conference.

Teacher: David, what happened on the test?
David: I dunno.
Teacher: Did you study?
David: Yeah—a lot.
Teacher: A lot?
David: Well, some.
Teacher: Then why did you do so poorly on the test?
David: You asked the wrong questions.
Teacher: What do you mean?
David: Teachers are all alike. They ask dumb questions.
Teacher: I expect you to know the material.
David: I still think the test was dumb.
Teacher: David, you're a bright young man.
David: Yeah? Then why did I flunk your test?

Teacher: I think you don't really apply yourself.
David: I think it's because the questions you ask are dumb.
Teacher: All right, what should be on the test?
David: Better questions.
Teacher: Well, then . . . you're getting a second chance. This time you will write the test questions.
David: Me? What do you mean?
Teacher: Sure. I want you to write five good test questions.
David: Five?
Teacher: If you studied at all it shouldn't be too hard.
David: But, uh, I don't think I have the time.
Teacher: Maybe you'll have time in summer school.
David: In other words, I don't have a choice.
Teacher: David, I want to help you but you've got to show some effort. Put on your thinking cap.
David: Uhhhh, I don't think I have one of those.
Teacher: Start writing . . .

Car Trouble

A woman has taken her car into the shop for repair. The car is up on the hoist, and she and the mechanic are looking up at the underside of the car.

Mechanic: Hmmmm. This doesn't look good.
Customer: What do you mean?
Mechanic: Just look at that part.
Customer: Look at what?
Mechanic: Right there.
Customer: How can I tell?
Mechanic: That's my point.
Customer: What is?
Mechanic: It's in such bad shape, it's unrecognizable.
Customer: But I don't know what it is supposed to look like.
Mechanic: Not likc that. It should look like this one.
Customer: How in the world am I supposed to know if you are giving me the facts?
Mechanic: I'm not giving you a line, lady. Honesty is our middle name.
Customer: I knew I should have had my husband do this.
Mechanic: Yep, it's the end of the road for that part. I'm surprised it's lasted this long.
Customer: I already told you, I don't know about car parts. I don't know what it is supposed to look like. And you're not being very helpful.
Mechanic: But it's as clear as the nose on your face.
Customer: To me, it's as clear as mud!
Mechanic: Okay, lady, you don't need to get huffy about it.
Customer: Don't "Lady" me, mister. Who is in charge here?
Mechanic: George.
Customer: I'm going to give him a piece of my mind.
Mechanic: He's out to lunch.

Customer: Well, he's not the only one!
Mechanic: Take it easy, lady. You're getting a little hot under the hood.
Customer: I've had enough. Give me my keys.
Mechanic: Suit yourself.
Customer: I'm out of here.
Mechanic: Okay. But, don't you want me to lower your car first?

Chores

Joe and his mother have a discussion about his jobs around the house.

Mom: Joe, we need to talk.
Joe: Mom, I'm up here.
Mom: Come down here. Now!
Joe: What's up?
Mom: You haven't done your chores all week.
Joe: It's been a really busy week, Mom.
Mom: You didn't mow the lawn.
Joe: I told you, the mower isn't working.
Mom: Your father told you two days ago that he fixed it. I heard him tell you.
Joe: I probably forgot. I've had lots of things happening. My life is very dynamic.
Mom: Not so dynamic that you can't find time to play on the computer and hang out with your friends.
Joe: Mom, none of my friends have to do stuff like that around the house. I'm the only one. No one uses the word "chores" any more.
Mom: Chores, jobs, duties—I don't care what you call them. As long as you live in this house, young man, you'll have them.
Joe: I can't believe it.
Mom: And, you didn't take the garbage to the curb yesterday, so the garbage truck missed it.
Joe: I was too busy. I was studying for my math test.
Mom: The garbage truck will pick it up today for an extra fee. Have your money ready.
Joe: Ah, Mom! I can't afford that.
Mom: And, if you don't mow by this afternoon, Spencer next door will do it.
Joe: He charges way too much!
Mom: And you'll pay it!
Joe: Mom, that's unfair!
Mom: Joseph, you have only a few jobs around here. We're tired of you not pulling your weight.
Joe: But, I'm going over to Phil's house in an hour.
Mom: Your plans have changed
Joe: What will I tell the guys?
Mom: Tell them you've decided that it's time you take some responsibility around the house. Tell them that you want to demonstrate respect and appreciation for your family and our home.
Joe: Huh?
Mom: Just mow the lawn . . .

Radio Show

Bob has a collection of old radio show recordings he enjoys. Jen isn't interested in them.

Jen: Are you still listening to that old program?
Bob: Sure. It's great.
Jen: Why don't you watch TV like other men your age?
Bob: And miss a night with Lamont Cranston?
Jen: Who?
Bob: He's the guy who turns into "The Shadow."
Jen: For crying out loud! How many times have you listened to that old thing?
Bob: Plenty. Listen to this part. It's from my favorite episode, "Carnival of Death."
Jen: All right. The sound effects are pretty good. And his laugh is creepy.
Bob: "Heh-heh-heh. Who knows what evil lurks in the hearts of men?"
Jen: Yes, I know, "The Shadow knows." That gives me the willies.
Bob: It's supposed to do that. It's suspenseful. People used to sit glued to the radio listening to these old programs and eating popcorn.
Jen: I prefer my popcorn in front of the TV.
Bob: Why don't you sit down and listen for a little while.
Jen: I've got things to do.
Bob: That's the beauty of radio shows. You can listen to them while you're doing something else.
Jen: I've got better things to do than to listen to some ancient ghost story on the radio.
Bob: You're not that busy! Stop a minute and use your imagination.
Jen: All right. I'm imagining—that you made dinner. That's really stretching the old imagination.
Bob: I surrender. Never mind.
Jen: Good. Now, what's going on in the garage?
Bob: What do you mean?
Jen: There it is again. Did you hear it? Go see what it is.
Bob: Sure. Lucky for me that I can "cloud men's minds" so they can't see me.
Jen: I'm serious. Just go out there and see.
Bob: Okay.
Jen: What is it?
Bob: Heh-heh-heh. Come out here and see for yourself.
Jen: That's not funny.
Bob: It's just the wind coming in under the garage door. It's blowing a few leaves around the garage. I've got to fix that.
Jen: That's all?
Bob: Yep. No boogeyman.
Jen: Good.
Bob: So, what are you going to do now?
Jen: Maybe I'll listen to your radio show with you.
Bob: You will? I'll be darned! You know, you're pretty unpredictable.
Jen: Who knows what lurks in the hearts of men? Or women?

Accident

At the scene of a minor car accident the two drivers decide how to handle the situation.

Driver 1: Why don't you watch where you're going?
Driver 2: Me?
Driver 1: If you hadn't run that stop sign this wouldn't have happened. It's all your fault.
Driver 2: What do you mean, my fault?
Driver 1: Come on, admit it! You caused this. Now give me your name and address.
Driver 2: I have no intention of giving you that information.
Driver 1: Fine. The cops can do that. I'm calling them now. Stay right where you are.
Driver 2: Wait a minute. Don't call the police. It isn't necessary. Look, there's no great damage to either car.
Driver 1: Forget it. I'm calling the cops.
Driver 2: We can settle this ourselves and there won't be any traffic tickets given.
Driver 1: Why worry about a ticket if it wasn't your fault?
Driver 2: If I get another ticket they'll drop my insurance.
Driver 1: Oh-ho! So you've been in a few accidents.
Driver 2: Well, yes . . . but if you hadn't been here, this one wouldn't have happened.
Driver 1: Oh, that makes a lot of sense. I'm calling the cops.
Driver 2: Let's settle and get out of here.
Driver 1: No way! People like you shouldn't be allowed to drive. I want justice here. The world needs to be protected from maniacs like you.
Driver 2: Look, I'll pay for everything, and I'll give you $100 cash.
Driver 1: You can't buy me off like that. You're a menace to society. They should put you away.
Driver 2: I'll give you 500 bucks. That will easily cover the scratch on your bumper and put 300 bucks in your pocket.
Driver 1: I can't believe this. It's my duty as a good citizen to see you get your just desserts. Where is a cop when you need one?
Driver 2: All right, here's my last offer. I'll give you $1,000 cash. I hardly even touched your bumper. You have everything to gain. Here's the cash.
Driver 1: Money can't buy everything, you know. Hey, is that a $1,000.00 bill? I've never seen one before.
Driver 2: Yes, it's real. Take a good look.
Driver 1: Hmmm . . . It looks like the real thing.
Driver 2: Believe me, it is. Keep it.
Driver 1: That is tempting. Let me think a second. Hmmm. All right, I will keep it, even though it's against my better judgment.
Driver 2: Thanks. Sorry for the inconvenience. I need to get going.
Driver 1: All right. But, don't let this happen again. I don't usually do this kind of thing, you know. You're lucky that you ran into a descent, forgiving guy like me. That doesn't happen every day, you know.

Fish Story

Jason and Phil have been fishing buddies for a long time. They usually tell the truth about their fishing trips. But, sometimes, one or the other stretches the truth a bit.

Jason: Have you been out lately?
Phil: Out where?
Jason: Out fishing.
Phil: Uh-huh.
Jason: You have? When?
Phil: This morning.
Jason: Today?
Phil: Uh-huh.
Jason: Why didn't you tell me?
Phil: I forgot.
Jason: Forgot! How could you forget?
Phil: I don't know.
Jason: You know I've been wanting to see that secret fishing hole of yours.
Phil: I know.
Jason: I know you know. So why didn't you call me?
Phil: If I took you to it, it wouldn't be a secret.
Jason: I wouldn't tell anyone.
Phil: Sure.
Jason: Really, I wouldn't.
Phil: Uh-huh.
Jason: Well, did you catch anything?
Phil: Yep.
Jason: You did? How many?
Phil: Four.
Jason: Wow! How big were they?
Phil: Oh, about like that.
Jason: That big! You're kidding!
Phil: Nope. Actually, one was a little bigger than that.
Jason: You're full of baloney.
Phil: Look, do you want proof?
Jason: Yeah.
Phil: Okay. Come on over for dinner tonight.
Jason: What are you having?
Phil: Well, it won't be buffalo steaks!
Jason: So, what are you having?
Phil: We're having fish, you ding-dong!
Jason: I still think you are pulling my leg.
Phil: Okay, stay at home and have macaroni and cheese for the third night in a row. I don't care.
Jason: Wait a minute. I believe that you caught some fish. What time is dinner?

Phil: Does that mean you're coming over?
Jason: Sure. I'm tired of macaroni. What time?
Phil: About six.
Jason: What should I bring?
Phil: Something to drink . . . and a steak knife.

Exercise Plan

Experts say exercise is important for people of all ages. When starting an exercise program, start gradually.

Sam: Ugh! Getting old isn't so great.
Jim: What do you mean?
Sam: My back is killing me. I get tired easily. It's no picnic.
Jim: You know what they say.
Sam: What's that?
Jim: Consider the alternative.
Sam: Can't you ever say something original? Something clever?
Jim: Just because your back hurts doesn't mean you get to take it out on me!
Sam: It's true! Everything you say is as old as the hills.
Jim: And twice as dusty?
Sam: There you go again. Oooh, my back!
Jim: Maybe you need a new exercise routine.
Sam: How can I do exercise if I hurt all the time?
Jim: I recently read about an exercise that might help.
Sam: I told you, I hurt too much to exercise.
Jim: It's supposed to build strength in your arms . . . probably in your back, too.
Sam: It will probably just break my back into two painful pieces.
Jim: You're supposed to do it three times a week. I do it. I think it's working.
Sam: You do it? All right. What is it?
Jim: You take a 5-pound potato sack in each hand.
Sam: Potato sacks? Okay. What's next?
Jim: Extend your arms straight out from your sides.
Sam: Two 5-pound sacks?
Jim: Yep. Hold them there for a full minute if you can. Then relax.
Sam: That's a lot of weight for that long.
Jim: Each day you'll find you can do it a little longer.
Sam: I'll be paralyzed!
Jim: After a couple of weeks, progress to 10-pound potato sacks.
Sam: Ten pounds?
Jim: Then, 50-pound sacks. Eventually, try to get to where you can lift 100-pound sacks in each hand for a full minute.
Sam: That's impossible! I'd be dead!
Jim: When you're confident, you go to the next level.

Sam: What's that?
Jim: You put a potato in each sack.
Sam: What?! Why, you . . .
Jim: Ahhh, ha, ha, ha. Was that clever enough for you?
Sam: I should have known! I'm going to strangle you.
Jim: You'll have to catch me first.
Sam: You better start running, buddy.
Jim: What about your back? I thought you were in terrible pain.
Sam: Like I said, start running.
Jim: Hey, Hot Shot, you forgot all about the tremendous pain you were having! I guess laughter is the best medicine. Too bad I'm not very original. Ha, ha . . .

Computer Problem

Ted is using the computer that he and Joe share for their college classes.

Ted: Uh-oh.
Joe: What's up?
Ted: Uhh. I'm not sure.
Joe: What was the "uh-oh" about?
Ted: Just hang on a second . . . Oh, no!
Joe: What's wrong?
Ted: Oh, this can't be happening.
Joe: What do you mean?
Ted: It's gone. It's all gone. Everything! Erased!
Joe: That's impossible.
Ted: See for yourself. Oh, no! Why now?
Joe: But what about my term paper? It's due tomorrow.
Ted: I should have known when I heard that clicking sound.
Joe: Where's my term paper? I've been working on it for weeks!
Ted: You're not going to find it. This computer is history. So is everything in it. I can't believe this.
Joe: What? But my term paper is in there.
Ted: I'll say it slowly. The computer has crashed. Your term paper is toast.
Joe: Toast? My term paper can't be toast!
Ted: Luckily, I saved all my important projects on this memory device.
Joe: Yes! That's it! I don't have to worry. I saved my paper.
Ted: Where?
Joe: On the computer. I saved it in there.
Ted: You still don't get it, do you. And I've told you a dozen times.
Joe: What do you mean?
Ted: You've got to save important things outside the computer, like on this thing. It's a backup. So, if your computer crashes—like right now—you'll still have all your work.
Joe: I'll get it out of there.

Ted: Hitting the screen isn't going to help.
Joe: Ahhhhhhhhh
Ted: And banging on the keyboard won't fix it either. . . . Here, let me hit it.
Joe: I can't just let all that work go down the drain. I can't start all over.
Ted: Well . . . what are we going to do?
Joe: What about those computer guys at the store. Maybe they can fix it.
Ted: I hope you have a lot of money. It will be expensive.
Joe: I've got to do something. That was my best writing ever!
Ted: Maybe they can help, but I doubt it.
Joe: Ohhhhhh. This is the worst! I'll never use a computer again.
Ted: You think so? How will you write your next term paper?
Joe: I don't know.
Ted: I suppose you could use pen and paper.
Joe: How does that work?
Ted: Never mind. Let's take this piece of junk to the computer store.

The Wise One Answers Life's Hard Questions

A man calls The Wise One call-in radio show for advice. He begins to wonder about the quality of the advice he is getting.

Wise One: Hello. This is The Wise One here to answer life's hard questions.
Caller: Hello, Wise One. I have a couple of questions.
Wise One: Go ahead.
Caller: My doctor tells me to eat less and exercise more.
Wise One: What for?
Caller: He says I should exercise more to raise my heart rate, and I will become healthier.
Wise One: Look, your heart is good for only so many beats.
Caller: What?
Wise One: Everything wears out eventually, doesn't it? If you speed up your heart rate, you'll bite the dust sooner.
Caller: Are you sure about that? I read that . . .
Wise One: Think of it this way, if you want your car to last longer, do you drive it faster?
Caller: No, but I don't think that's the same.
Wise One: It's only logical. If you want to live longer, take a nap.
Caller: I never thought of it like that.
Wise One: That's why they call me The Wise One.
Caller: I have another question.
Wise One: Shoot.
Caller: My doctor says I should cut down on red meat and eat more fruits and vegetables.
Wise One: What for?
Caller: He says I'm eating too much fat. But, I sure like eating steak!
Wise One: That doesn't make sense. Obviously your doctor hasn't thought this out very well. And, it doesn't take a rocket scientist.

Caller: What do you mean?
Wise One: Look, beef is from cattle, right?
Caller: Right.
Wise One: Cattle eat grass, hay, and grain. Right?
Caller: Yeah.
Wise One: So when you eat a steak you're actually eating vegetables and grains. They're just in a different form.
Caller: Hmmmm. I don't think it works that way.
Wise One: It's simple arithmetic!
Caller: I really don't think it is that simple.
Wise One: Why make things so complicated?
Caller: But, I think I'm starting to understand where you're coming from.
Wise One: What do you mean?
Caller: Well, answer this. My doctor also tells me I should limit how much wine and beer I drink.
Wise One: Why would he say that? I think you should . . .
Caller: Let me guess. I bet you're going to say I should drink more wine and beer because they're made out of fruits and grains.
Wise One: Exactly! I told you it doesn't take a rocket scientist.
Caller: Wise One, I'm not too sure about your logic.
Wise One: You're welcome. And feel free to ask The Wise One any of life's hard questions at any time.
Caller: Gee, thanks, Wise One. But, don't hold your breath.

New Roommate

Tom thought he chose the right roommate. Now he thinks he made a bad decision.

Ray: Time to get up
Tom: Huh?
Ray: It's 6:30.
Tom: Who are . . . ?
Ray: Who? It's me. Your new roomy.
Tom: Yeah. I remember.
Ray: You said you had to get up at 6:30.
Tom: That's what my alarm is for.
Ray: I'm just helping you out.
Tom: What time is it?
Ray: 6:30.
Tom: Already? Ohhhh. I hardly slept.
Ray: Time to rise and shine.
Tom: I'm going back to sleep.
Ray: Toast?
Tom: What? Are you still here?

Ray: Do you want some toast?
Tom: No, I don't want toast. I'm going back to sleep.
Ray: Okay. Just thought you might want some breakfast.
Tom: Shut the door.
Ray: Vitamins.
Tom: What?
Ray: I said, "Vitamins."
Tom: What are you talking about?
Ray: Maybe you need some.
Tom: I don't need vitamins. Get out and be quiet!
Ray: I'm full of vitality in the morning. You know what they say. "The early bird gets the worm."
Tom: This is not working. You living here. With me.
Ray: Yeah, it's great. I love this place.
Tom: No! It's not working.
Ray: This is for you—a tall glass of my special morning elixir.
Tom: What are you yakking about?
Ray: It's my own recipe. Tofu. Seaweed. Organic herbs.
Tom: I've had it! You've been here two days. That's two days too many.
Ray: But, we're just getting used to each other.
Tom: No. I know enough about you. We're incompatible.
Ray: You're jumping the gun. It can work. You'll see.
Tom: No, it can't. You're making me crazy. I don't like you.
Ray: You'll learn to like me.
Tom: No, I won't. And you don't like me. You just don't know it yet.
Ray: Man, you wake up really cranky!
Tom: I wake up just fine!
Ray: Maybe you're low on iron.
Tom: Stop talking!
Ray: Take some deep breaths. In comes the good air, out goes the bad. It works wonders.
Tom: Get out! Now! I'm going back to sleep. You're moving out by tomorrow.
Ray: Man, you certainly got up on the wrong side of the bed!

Goddess

Max talks his friend Ted into helping him arrange a date with a beautiful classmate.

Ted: Hi! How's it going?
Max: Pretty good. How did that test go?
Ted: Who knows? It wasn't too bad.
Max: I hate everything about that class, except . . .
Ted: Except Leslie, the most gorgeous woman on the planet?
Max: How did you know?
Ted: I'm not blind! Do you think you're the only one? She drives every guy in school nuts.

Max: I wonder if she would go out with me?
Ted: She could go out with anyone. Why would she go out with you?
Max: She isn't going out with anyone right now, is she?
Ted: I don't think so.
Max: What a goddess! Notice how every one just stares when she walks by?
Ted: She won't go out with you. You're too ugly.
Max: Hey, next to you I look like Cary Grant.
Ted: Who's that?
Max: Some dead actor my Mom talks about.
Ted: You're still too ugly for her. She's incredible!
Max: Hmmm. There must be a way. Any ideas?
Ted: Plastic surgery.
Max: What?
Ted: You'll need to get your face fixed.
Max: Very funny. Come on, help me figure this out.
Ted: Okay, okay.
Max: Who do we know who knows her?
Ted: My sister, Tammy, has her in gym.
Max: Does Tammy talk to her?
Ted: She hasn't said much about her.
Max: We have to figure out a way for Tammy to get to know her. Then, invite her over to the house or something.
Ted: It won't be easy.
Max: Why not?
Ted: You know Tammy. The first thing she'll say is, "What's in it for me?"
Max: Tell her anything. Right now Leslie doesn't even know I'm alive. I don't have anything to lose.
Ted: I guess you're right.
Max: I can see it now. Leslie will be dazzled by my charm. Mesmerized by my wit.
Ted: Oh, please.
Max: I wonder if she likes a man with a mustache.
Ted: A mustache? You? Where are you going to buy one?
Max: Ha-ha. Will you talk with Tammy tonight?
Ted: I guess so.
Max: Good! A week from now Leslie will be throwing herself at me.
Ted: She'll probably throw up.
Max: We'll travel to Hawaii.
Ted: I'm getting sick.
Max: I wonder what our children will look like?
Ted: Probably like Cary Grant does right now.

New School

Kari and her mother moved from a small town to a city. She is unhappy with her new school.

Mom: Kari? Is that you?
Kari: Yeah.
Mom: I thought you would be home sooner.
Kari: I walked home.
Mom: Did you miss the bus?
Kari: No. I just felt like walking.
Mom: Are you feeling all right?
Kari: I guess so. But, I really wish we were back home.
Mom: This is our home now, Honey.
Kari: This isn't home to me. I want to go back to Idaho.
Mom: But, Honey . . .
Kari: I don't belong here.
Mom: We've only been here a week. You like our new house, don't you?
Kari: Yes. But I hate school.
Mom: It's only your first day.
Kari: I still hate it.
Mom: What's the problem?
Kari: Everything. It's too big. I don't know anybody. I hate it!
Mom: Not much like Idaho, is it.
Kari: No. I couldn't even get my locker open! And I was lost all day.
Mom: Oh, Kari, it's bound to get better.
Kari: What's the use? I don't know what to do.
Mom: Can you talk with a teacher? Or, make some kind of plan?
Kari: What do you mean?
Mom: Instead of being sad, figure out what to do.
Kari: How do I do that?
Mom: Let's see. You could go up to a group of girls in one of your classes and say, "Hi, I'm new around here, and I want to know what's going on!"
Kari: What? Are you kidding?
Mom: That would be a way to break the ice.
Kari: I can't believe it! They'd laugh me right out of the school!
Mom: It's worth a try.
Kari: Oh, right. "I'm new around here and I want to know what's going on."
Mom: I think it's a good idea.
Kari: Oh, Mother! I would never say anything that stupid to anyone! Parents just don't understand.
Mom: It's better than not doing anything, isn't it?
Kari: Whatever! I'll make my own plan, thank you.
Mom: Like what?
Kari: I don't know yet. Maybe I'll ask someone to help me with my locker first.
Mom: That sounds like a good start.

Kari: Did you really think I would say something that ridiculous?
Mom: Why not? I said something like that when I was young and started at a new school.
Kari: That was at the turn of the last century, Mother.
Mom: Not quite, but I did meet some new people.
Kari: They probably just thought you were really strange.
Mom: Making a plan always works better than stewing over something.
Kari: Maybe. We'll see. Well, talking with you has helped a little.
Mom: That's wonderful. How?
Kari: Now I definitely know what NOT to do tomorrow! Thanks, Mom.

Second Opinion

A woman goes to a doctor to get a second opinion about her diet.

Doctor: Hello. Mrs. Jones?
Patient: Yes.
Doctor: I'm Dr. Smith
Patient: It's nice to meet you.
Doctor: Now, I understand you are here for a second opinion.
Patient: That's right. I thought a doctor who was a woman would set things straight.
Doctor: Your records weren't sent to me.
Patient: I know. I didn't want you to have your mind made up before you saw me.
Doctor: What is the nature of your problem?
Patient: Can you guess?
Doctor: Does it have to do with your weight?
Patient: So you noticed?
Doctor: Indeed. You are quite overweight.
Patient: That's what my regular doctor told me. He's been concerned for a while.
Doctor: Then, you have discussed this with him?
Patient: Many times. He thinks I'm not following the diet he gave me.
Doctor: Tell me more.
Patient: Well, he gave me a booklet that said I should be eating foods from the basic food groups at every meal.
Doctor: Have you been following that advice?
Patient: I certainly have. To the letter.
Doctor: Then, what's the problem?
Patient: He says that I eat what I want to eat and that I'm not taking the diet seriously.
Doctor: Are those his exact words?
Patient: Something like that.
Doctor: And you don't agree?
Patient: Absolutely not!
Doctor: Well, what is a typical breakfast for you?
Patient: I like grains, so I start out with a few items from that food group. Usually three or four doughnuts. They're whole wheat, of course.

Doctor: Uh, that's how you start?

Patient: Of course, I can't ignore the other food groups! I have never liked fruit much, but I discovered fruit pies help me meet that requirement. So I usually have a piece or two of apple or cherry pie. Sometimes both. They say you can never get enough fruit.

Doctor: Doughnuts and pie?

Patient: Yes, and I include the dairy group here, too—two scoops of vanilla ice cream on the pie. It's like killing two birds with one stone. Know what I mean?

Doctor: I think I'm getting the picture. Did you say you eat like this every day?

Patient: You betcha! Just following the doctor's orders.

Doctor: Did you eat that much before following the diet your doctor gave you?

Patient: Are you kidding? My eating used to be completely out of control. Thank heaven I'm finally eating the right things now. Do you want to hear about the rest of my diet?

Doctor: I don't think I need to. I'm feeling full just listening to you.

Patient: Milk by itself is so bland, so to complete the dairy group, I usually have a milkshake.

Doctor: Somehow I knew that was coming.

Patient: You're a mind reader! I flavor the shake with hot fudge sauce. It really livens up an otherwise ho-hum drink.

Doctor: Oh, my! Well, from everything you've told me, I think that . . .

Patient: I'm not finished. I haven't even mentioned the meat group yet.

Doctor: But . . .

Patient: No, you've got to believe me when I say I do my best to eat from all the major food groups with hardly any snacking in between meals.

Doctor: In that case, go ahead. I'm on the edge of my seat!

Patient: Now, the meat requirement is kind of a tough one, but every morning I do my best to eat plenty of bacon and sausage. Sometimes I'm so full I can hardly get out of the chair to freshen up my milkshake.

Doctor: Please, stop!

Patient: And by the time I've finished with breakfast, lunchtime is just around the corner.

Doctor: You don't need to say another word.

Patient: Don't you want to hear what I have to go through at lunchtime?

Doctor: No. I've heard enough. Mrs. Jones, you are eating way too much. If you don't reduce your intake by hundreds of calories each day, you will certainly experience some serious health problems in the very near future.

Patient: What do you mean? I've been following the doctor's orders— the food groups, I mean.

Doctor: Surely, you realize that you are consuming so much fat and sugar every day that you will continue to gain weight.

Patient: That's what my regular doctor said! And I thought I was doing so well with those food groups. I should have known it. You doctors are all alike. I think you're all in cahoots!

Doctor: Mrs. Jones, I want to help you.

Patient: I don't believe you. No matter what I do, the doctor says it's wrong.

Doctor: Please, Mrs. Jones, let's discuss this some more.

Patient: No. I've heard enough. I'm leaving!

Doctor: Where are you going?

Patient: Out to find someone who really listens to me—someone who isn't so critical. I'm getting a third opinion!

"Write and Practice Your Own Dialogues" Form

Goal area or target skills to be addressed in this dialogue:

____

____

Title: ____________________________________

____

Situation: __________________________________

____

Speaker #1 ________________________________

Speaker #2 ________________________________

Speaker #1 ________________________________

Speaker #2 ________________________________

Speaker #1 ________________________________

Speaker #2 ________________________________

Speaker #1 ________________________________

Speaker #2 ________________________________

Speaker #1 ________________________________

Speaker #2 ________________________________

9

Contrastive Stress Drills

In *Voice and Articulation Drillbook,* Fairbanks (1960) demonstrated critical differences among consonants and among vowels and diphthongs through extensive use of contrastive minimal pairs. In addition, he described a therapeutic exercise using sentences that " . . . call for shifts of stress to each word in turn" (p. 161). This exercise incorporating shifts in stress is known as contrastive stress drill.

Notice the question-answer format of the following contrastive stress drill when the sentence, "I can do it," is spoken and the italicized words are stressed in turn, first by the clinician in the stimulus question, and then by the client in the response.

Question-Answer Format of Contrastive Stress Drills

Stimulus	**Clinician's stimulus questions with the stressed word *italicized***	**Client's responses showing alternating stress with the stressed word *italicized***
I can do it	"The sentence is, 'I can do it.' Say it."	"I can do it."
	"*Who* can do it?"	"*I* can do it."
	"You *can't* do it?"	"I *can* do it."
	"You can *eat* it?"	"I can *do* it."
	"You can do *what*?"	"I can do *it*."

The meaning of the sentence, "I can do it," changes when a particular word is stressed, but more importantly, the speaker presumably pays additional attention to a particular word, prepares for it, and executes it with louder voice, longer duration, and definitive articulatory precision. In this chapter contrastive stress drills are directed toward precise speech-sound production.

Wertz, LaPointe, and Rosenbek (1991) thoroughly discuss the application of contrastive stress drill in their classic text, *Apraxia of*

Speech in Adults: The Disorder and Its Management. They examine and refine the use of contrastive stress as a therapy technique for apraxia of speech, and conclude, "The contrastive stress drill may be one of the most potent techniques for stabilizing apraxic articulation and improving prosodic profiles" (p. 260). Although they limit their comments about the effectiveness of contrastive stress drill to therapy for apraxia of speech, their observations and rationale for why it is a useful and successful technique seem intuitively applicable to numerous speech and language therapy targets and populations. It is a technique that can be utilized with the majority of stimuli presented in previous chapters.

A contrastive stress drill for any given client should be developed according to rules (Wertz et al., 1991). All are essential and they are derived from a particular speaker's needs and what he can and cannot produce verbally. One of the prerequisites for engaging a client in contrastive stress drill is that the target of the exercise should be one that the client can actually produce or at least approximate some of the time. The drill itself cannot make a speech behavior appear when the speaker has little or no control over its production. If the client cannot produce a particular speech sound, Wertz et al. remind us that an exercise focusing on stress may need to follow treatment methods such as imitation ("Watch and listen; now you do it"), phonetic placement (Van Riper & Irwin, 1958; Vaughn & Clark, 1979; Young & Hawk, 1955), phonetic derivation (Van Riper & Irwin, 1958), and other techniques.

Why does contrastive stress drill work as a therapeutic technique for apraxia of speech? Wertz et al. (1991, p. 265) cite Kent (1976, p. 89) who wrote that rhythm acts as a kind of "substratum for virtually all perceptual and motor activities." Wertz et al. (1991, p. 264) state, "The contrastive stress drill may provide a stress-rhythm substratum that, for the apraxic patient, resembles the rhythmic basis of normal motor speech control and one that 'supports' or even 'summons' articulatory movements." They go on to say, (pp. 264–265):

"Regardless of why a contrastive stress drill works, it has advantages in addition to improving intelligibility. First, it adds variety, and apraxia of speech drills cry out for variety. Second, it resembles more normal conversation, because it is a series of questions and answers rather than a series of imitations. Finally, it moves the patient toward carryover, because it is more like what people do when they talk. No doubt the second and third interact; because the patient is practicing answers in the clinic, answers come easier outside."

In the following scenario of a contrastive stress drill of a minimal contrast pair with word-initial /l/ and /n/, the client can produce /n/ all of the time, but produces /l/ imprecisely much of the time. Moving from simple-to-complex responses, the clinician may first plan for the client to respond with a single word, as in #1 and #2, until accurate performance meets a certain criterion, then advance to a two-word response, as in #3, and possibly followed by longer responses, as in #4–#6.

A Contrastive Stress Drill of Minimal Pairs with Word-Initial /l/ and /n/

Minimal pair stimulus	Clinician's stimulus questions with stressed word *italicized*	Client's responses with stressed word *italicized*
knee - Lee	"*Knee*?"	"*Lee*!"
need - lead	"*Need*?"	"*Lead*!"
niece - lease	"Is the word *niece*?"	"No, *lease*!"
Nick - lick	"Is the word *Nick*?"	"The word is *lick*!"
knit - lit	"Is the word *knit*?"	"Not knit, *lit*!"
nag - lag	"Is the word *nag*?"	"Not nag, Jack, *lag*!"

When developing a contrastive stress drill for a client, the particular question-answer format and target of the exercise should be understood by the client. Otherwise, the cognitive requirements of trying to figure out the format may be overwhelming and move the focus of the exercise away from the speech-sound drill. Most aspects of a contrastive stress exercise can be modified as needed. For example, if stressing each word of a phrase or sentence becomes too cumbersome, odd, or difficult in any way, the clinician might consider presenting the question of the drill so that only particular words are stressed, such as the last word of a three-word phrase.

In the following scenario, the client produces the word-initial /f/ consistently, but most of the time he only approximates /s/ with occasional target productions. The target of the contrastive stress drills moves from the word with the unstable /s/ to the word with the stable /f/ sound, then back again. Note the additional words in the clinician's questions and in the client's responses. The /s/ remains the only target in the expected response; the client can accurately produce the other sounds in the longer response. If speech sounds that are not directly addressed in this drill are somewhat unstable in the client's repertoire, for example, final /ʃ/ in "sick fish," the clinician decides whether to delete that stimulus or keep it to increase the complexity of the task.

A Contrastive Stress Drill for Word-Initial /s/ and /f/ in Two-Word Phrases

Phrases contrasting word-initial /s/ and /f/	**Clinician's stimulus with stressed words *italicized***	**Client's response with stressed word *italicized***
some food	"*No* food?"	"*Some* food"
	"*Heavy* food?"	"*Some* food"
	"Some *baloney*?"	"Some *food*"
	"Some *car parts*?"	"Some *food*"
	"*Cat* food?"	"*Some* food"
sword fight	"*Fist* fight?"	"*Sword* fight"
	"*Pillow* fight?	"*Sword* fight"
	"Sword *duel*?"	"Sword *fight*"
	"*Jell-o fight*?"	"*Sword* fight"
	"Sword *sharpener*?"	"Sword *fight*"
sick fish	"*Healthy* fish?"	"*Sick* fish"
	"Sick *oyster*?"	"Sick *fish*"
	"*Funny* fish?"	"*Sick* fish"
	"Sick *squid*?"	"Sick *fish*"
	"*Comatose* fish?"	"*Sick* fish"

The following scenario of contrastive stress drill highlights the /r/ sound in sentences. The clinician modifies or deletes sentences that are too long or that contain too many occurrences of the target sound that cause the client excessive frustration or impede practice or progress.

A Contrastive Stress Drill Focusing on the /r/ Sound

Sentences with the /r/ sound	**Clinician's stimulus with stressed words *italicized***	**Client's response with stressed word *italicized***
I'm really rich	"*Who's* really rich?"	"*I'm* really rich."
	"You're *kind of* rich?"	"I'm *really* rich."
	"You're really *poor*?"	"I'm really *rich*."
It rolled across the room	"It *slid* across the room?"	"It *rolled* across the room."
	"It rolled *around* the room?"	"It rolled *across* the room."
	"It rolled across the *floor*?"	"It rolled across the *room*"

SUGGESTIONS FOR DEVELOPING, USING, AND MODIFYING CONTRASTIVE STRESS DRILLS

- At first, require simple one-word and two-word responses that address the client's speech target. Consider his or her speech production capabilities and the cognitive-language requirements of the entire task before expecting the client's production of the speech target in longer, more complex responses. Design the task so the client is able to articulate all or most of the non-target speech sounds in the expected response.
- With success, the complexity of the expected speech response may be increased in any number of ways, such as increasing the length of response required, multiple occurrences of a particular speech sound in a response, occurrence of two different speech targets in a single response, and removal of printed cues.
- The purpose of these contrastive stress drills is for a client to practice particular speech targets. It is not to challenge the client's memory for sentences (although contrastive stress drill can be an excellent technique for addressing memory for sentences and grammatical aspects of spoken language). Assuming the client has adequate reading ability, provide the printed stimulus for him to refer to during speech practice. If the client's reading ability or visual acuity is compromised, the expected response should be short.
- The client is encouraged to listen to and study the clinician's articulatory and prosodic model, as well as to listen to and feel his own speech productions. The clinician's slow-paced and contemplative presentation of a stimulus question may help the client to respond with a slower than usual, contemplative response.
- Using Base-10 Response Forms as described in Chapter 10 has many advantages for planning and keeping track of progress in therapy with contrastive stress drills.
- Contrastive stress drills can be an excellent therapy technique, but it can be very demanding and become tedious for both the client and clinician. Use a variety of therapy techniques and therapy materials in any given session.

- The speech-language pathologist may want to give the client material for speech practice outside the therapy session. For contrastive stress drills, home practice requires that the client have an informed, able, and congenial partner to present the stimulus questions. The form entitled, "Practice Stressing the Italicized Words" on the final pages of this chapter may be helpful for planning practice at home. The clinician writes stimuli in the left column labeled, "The words are . . . " The stimulus questions for the client's partner are written in the middle column with the stressed words italicized. The expected responses of the client are entitled "My Responses" written in the right column with the stressed words italicized. Modify the directions at the top of the sheet as needed.
  Humor helps.

"PRACTICE STRESSING THE ITALICIZED WORDS" FORM

Directions: The client and the partner practice this stress drill by reading through the example, "Call the cops." The key phrase is in the left column under "The words are . . . " The partner asks a question in the middle column, stressing the italicized word. The client says the response written in the right column, stressing the italicized word. Suggestions: Don' rush. Enjoy it.

The words are . . .	**Partner's Questions**	**My Responses**
Example: Call the cops	*See* the cops?	*Call* the cops
	Call *those* cops?	Call *the* cops
	Call the *Pizza Palace*?	Call the *cops*
1. The words are . . .	**Partner's Questions**	**My Responses**
2. The words are . . .	**Partner's Questions**	**My Responses**
3. The words are . . .	**Partner's Questions**	**My Responses**

4. The words are . . .	Partner's Questions	My Responses
5. The words are . . .	**Partner's Questions**	**My Responses**
6. The words are . . .	**Partner's Questions**	**My Responses**
7. The words are . . .	**Partner's Questions**	**My Responses**
8. The words are . . .	**Partner's Questions**	**My Responses**

9. The words are . . .	Partner's Questions	My Responses
10. The words are . . .	**Partner's Questions**	**My Responses**

10

Keeping on Track in Therapy with Base-10 Response Forms

In this book the author's intention has been to provide practical speech therapy practice material for speech-language pathologists. It is not intended to instruct clinicians about how to do therapy. Yet, a particular tool, the Base-10 Response Form (LaPointe, 1977; 1985, 1991), has been successfully used throughout the years and continues to help clinicians plan, organize, and stay on track in therapy. It is a convenient, versatile, and powerful instrument well-suited for measuring and documenting progress in therapy.

At first glance, the Base-10 Response Form appears as a simple scoring and charting form, but it is actually an elegant method of specifying stimuli and scoring and plotting performance on speech-language management tasks, and it serves as a basis for making important decisions about therapy. The Base-10 Response Form has application in everyday therapy as well as in single study research. Dr. LaPointe has granted permission to all speech-language clinicians to use Base-10 Response Forms to augment the speech and language treatment they provide, and he has permitted inclusion of a blank Base-10 Response Form (Figure 10–1) in this manual (J. E. Thomas, personal communication, March 13, 2007). The author is grateful and indebted to Dr. LaPointe.

If the clinician is not already familiar with the Base-10 Response Form and the programmed approach to therapy it supports, it is important to understand what the form is not and what it does not do. The Base-10 Response Form is not a tally sheet for recording moment-to-moment responses during a therapy session. And, using the Base-10 form does not constitute therapy. Rather, the Base-10 Response Form is a method of systematically sampling and documenting how a client is performing and progressing at a particular speech-language task over a period of time.

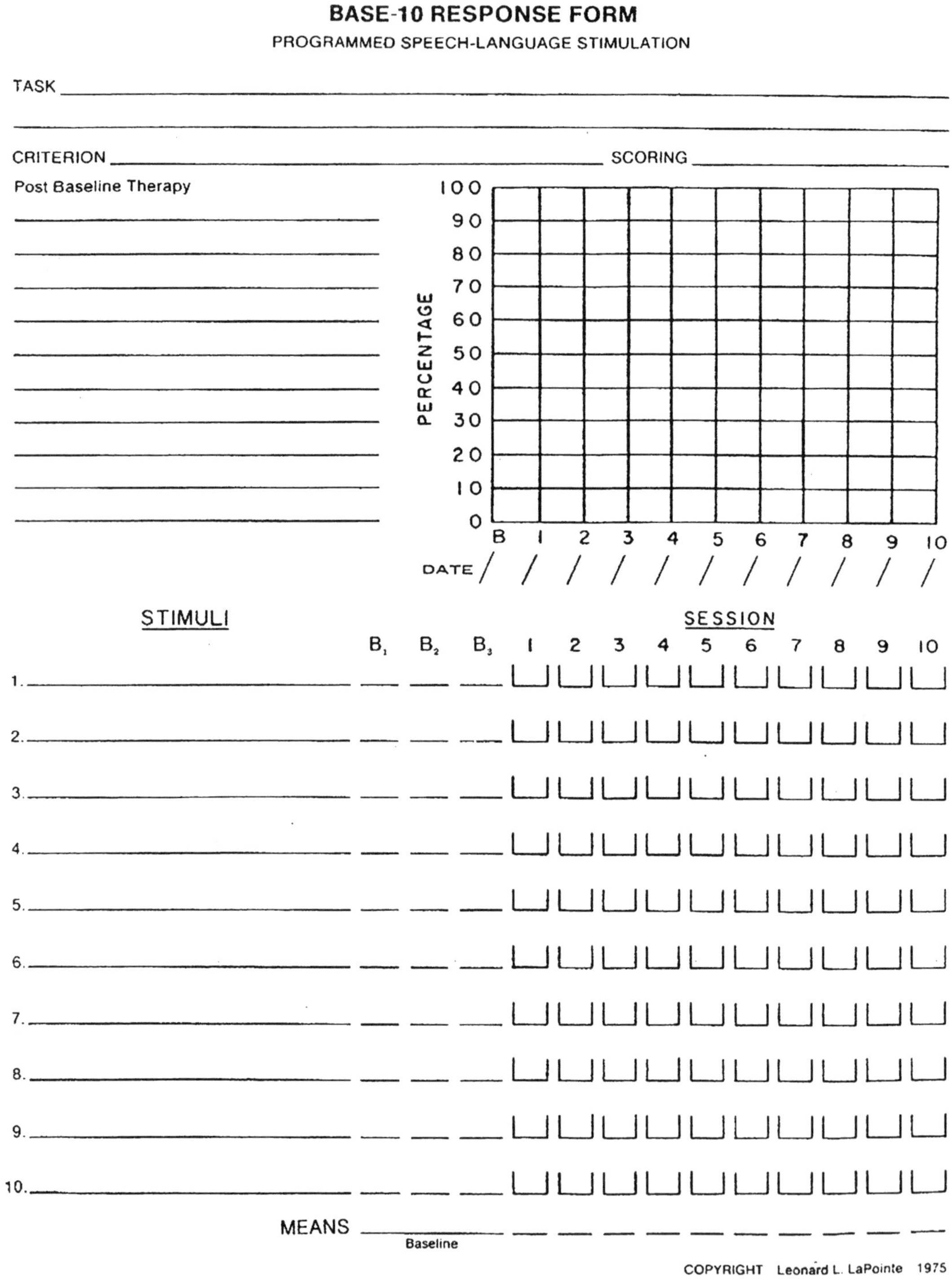

BASE-10 RESPONSE FORM

PROGRAMMED SPEECH-LANGUAGE STIMULATION

TASK ______

CRITERION ______ SCORING ______

Post Baseline Therapy

PERCENTAGE

100 90 80 70 60 50 40 30 20 10 0

B 1 2 3 4 5 6 7 8 9 10

DATE / / / / / / / / / / /

STIMULI

SESSION

	B_1	B_2	B_3	1	2	3	4	5	6	7	8	9	10
1.													
2.													
3.													
4.													
5.													
6.													
7.													
8.													
9.													
10.													

MEANS ______ (Baseline)

COPYRIGHT Leonard L. LaPointe 1975

Figure 10–1. Base-10 Response Form. Reprinted by permission from Base-10 Programmed Stimulation: Task Specification, Scoring, and Plotting Performance in Aphasia Therapy by L. L. LaPointe. *Journal of Speech and Hearing Disorders*, *42*, 90–105. Copyright 1977 by American Speech-Language-Hearing Association. All rights reserved.

THE BASE-10 RESPONSE FORM—IN A NUTSHELL

The Base-10 Response Form was first developed for the "... purpose of improving the focus and convenience of daily treatment" (LaPointe, 1991, p. 2.), primarily for aphasia therapy. Nevertheless, the format is sufficiently adaptable to many speech-language targets unrelated to aphasia. Included here is a general summary of the Base-10 approach to measuring progress of skill acquisition, with some information taken from the Base-10 Response Form Revised Manual (LaPointe, 1991), which is no longer in print. Clinicians are encouraged to refer to LaPointe (1977, 1985) for thorough background, descriptions and numerous examples of therapeutic applications for the Base-10 Response Form, including examples of speech, verbal expression, auditory comprehension, reading, and writing tasks.

The components of the Base-10 Response Form are straightforward. Refer to the blank form in Figure 10-1.

Select a Therapeutic Task

A therapeutic task is selected and written on the top lines of the Base-10 Response Form. Task selection is based on the results and analysis of the client's speech and language evaluation. It is likely there will be several therapy tasks in each session addressing several therapy goals. A separate Base-10 form is used to sample behaviors toward each therapeutic task.

Determining Criterion and Selecting Stimuli

Criteria for achieving the task goal are written at the upper left of the form. Criteria may vary from task to task, but a common level of performance expectation before advancement to the next level of many tasks is 80% to 90% accuracy over three consecutive therapy sessions. Stimuli are listed on the lines at the left of the Base-10 form. These are 10 specific items such as phonetic symbols, a list of particular words, phrases, or sentences, and so forth.

Scoring

Scoring for the task is specified near the upper right corner of the form. Simple systems such as a plus-or-minus scoring for correct/incorrect responses are easy to apply, and performance on some speech and language tasks does not require more specificity or sensitivity. Other clinician-constructed scoring methods can be devised that account for a degree of approximation to the target. Appendix 10-A presents several simple scoring systems and conversions of scores to percentages for charting on the Base-10 Response Form, but usually the clinician can adapt his or her preferred method of scoring to the Base-10 format, including more complex systems such as the 1-to-15 multidimensional scoring system of the Porch Index of Communicative Ability (PICA) (Porch, 1981).

Baseline Performance and Post-Baseline Therapy

Baseline measurement is necessary prior to initiating therapy to determine the client's preintervention performance level on any given task. The Base-10 form provides space for three samplings of a client's performance on the task stimuli. They are marked B1, B2, and B3 located in the middle of the form. These baselines may be taken at three successive sessions or during a single session. Baseline performance on any task informs the clinician of what the intervention should be or, as LaPointe (1991, p. 6) describes it, "... the treatment package or the particular strategy selected for modifying the student or client's performance on the task." The details of the treatment package are written in the section labeled "Post Baseline Therapy" in the upper left of the Base-10 form. LaPointe (1991) states that the therapy plan does not need to be comprehensive, but it should be described with some specificity for continuity in presentation of stimuli, as well as for future reference. The post-baseline therapy plan should also include any changes in programming along the way, such as altered reinforcement schedules, modification of stimulus presentation, and other pertinent information. Again, it is this specificity and planning which are the foundations of Base-10 therapy that focus the clinician to stay on track across a number of therapy sessions.

Calculating and Graphing the Score

After the therapeutic intervention for a task, or whenever the clinician decides to sample performance during the session, the 10 stimulus sampling items for the task that are written on the Base-10 form are administered. Then the score for each item is entered in the column for that session, and the total mean score is calculated at the bottom of the Base-10 Response Form. The mean score is converted to a percentage, and the percentage is entered on the graph in the upper right of the form. The graph serves as a visual display of progress, or lack of it, over a period of 10 sessions. The graph is easily understood by the client, family members, and other professionals, and it is concrete evidence and basis for future clinical questions and decisions.

In analyzing the client's performance, the clinician may ask questions, such as, "Do I stay on the present course?" "If not, how should the task be modified?" If an aspect of the task requires modification, but the task is not substantially changed, the modifications can be made on the same Base-10 form by drawing a vertical line down through the graph and session number to indicate when one phase has ended and a new phase begins. Whether the modifications concern the criterion, scoring, sampling stimuli, or post-baseline therapy, they are written and dated in the designated areas on the Base-10 form.

It is particularly important to keep in mind points cited earlier concerning use of the Base-10 Response Form and the therapy approach incorporated in its design. First, utilizing the Base-10 Response Form may be a part of every therapy session, but it is neither a therapy technique in itself, nor does using it constitute therapy. Second, when treatment is organized with the Base-10 form, the clinician must make many or most of the decisions about a therapy task early in the process, although modification of all aspects is always possible. This level of decision-making may take more time and development than that required for other treatment planning and methods of data collection and analysis. Nevertheless, the more frequently clinicians use Base-10 Response Forms the more efficient they become at making these decisions and realize the rewards of well-thought-out and documented speech management.

Examples of Speech Tasks on Base-10 Response Forms

The following examples represent a variety of speech management tasks and scoring systems on Base-10 Response Forms presented at various stages in therapy.

Figure 10–2 displays a speech task developed for a client with mild aphasia and marked apraxia of speech. She consistently substituted /t/ for /k/ in the initial position of common consonant-vowel-consonant (CVC) words. She was able to produce /k/ in word-final positions some of the time. Because of this problem she was unable to say her name correctly, which she found very embarrassing. Baseline sampling over three consecutive sessions showed that she produced initial /k/ in 10 selected CVC words 0% of the time. A therapy approach was determined and written in the Post-Baseline Therapy section of the Base-10 Response Form.

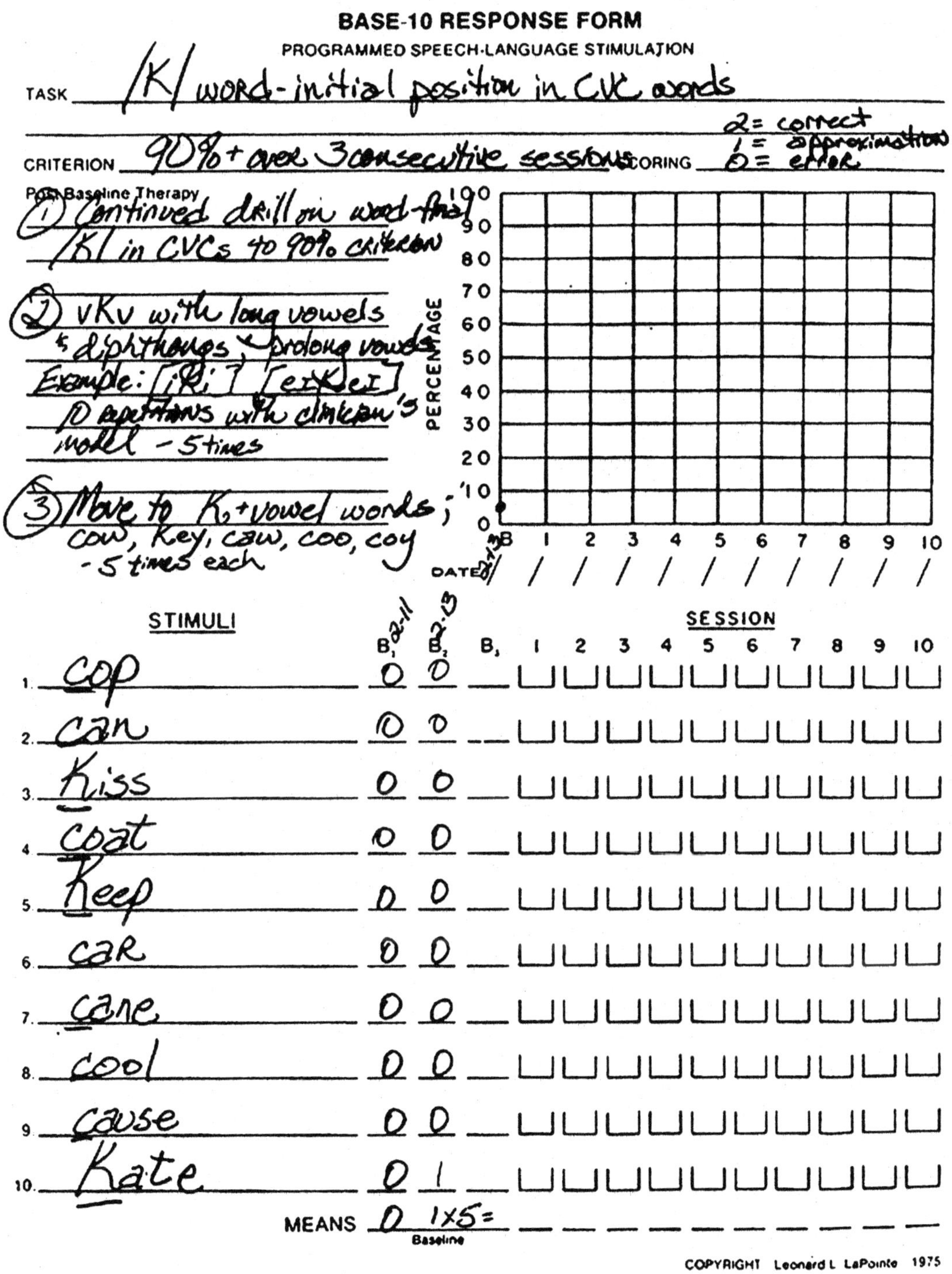

BASE-10 RESPONSE FORM

PROGRAMMED SPEECH-LANGUAGE STIMULATION

TASK /K/ word-initial position in CVC words

CRITERION 90%+ over 3 consecutive sessions

SCORING 2 = correct, 1 = approximation, 0 = error

Post-Baseline Therapy

① Continued drill on word-final /K/ in CVCs to 90% criterion

② VKV with long vowels & diphthongs, prolong vowels. Example: [iKi] [eɪKeɪ] 10 repetitions with clinician's model - 5 times

③ Move to K + vowel words; cow, key, caw, coo, coy - 5 times each

PERCENTAGE 100, 90, 80, 70, 60, 50, 40, 30, 20, 10, 0

B 1 2 3 4 5 6 7 8 9 10

DATE

STIMULI	B_1 (2-11)	B_2 (2-13)	B_3	SESSION 1–10
1. cop	0	0		
2. can	0	0		
3. kiss	0	0		
4. coat	0	0		
5. keep	0	0		
6. car	0	0		
7. cane	0	0		
8. cool	0	0		
9. cause	0	0		
10. Kate	0	1		
MEANS (Baseline)	0	1X5=		

COPYRIGHT Leonard L LaPointe 1975

Figure 10–2. Task: Production of /k/ word-initial position in CVC words.

Figure 10–3 illustrates a task for a patient with ataxic dysarthria of moderate severity who habitually telescoped polysyllabic words. He agreed to work at syllable-by-syllable production of words of increasing length. A consideration for an additional therapy task on a separate Base-10 form may have been to produce short common expressions composed

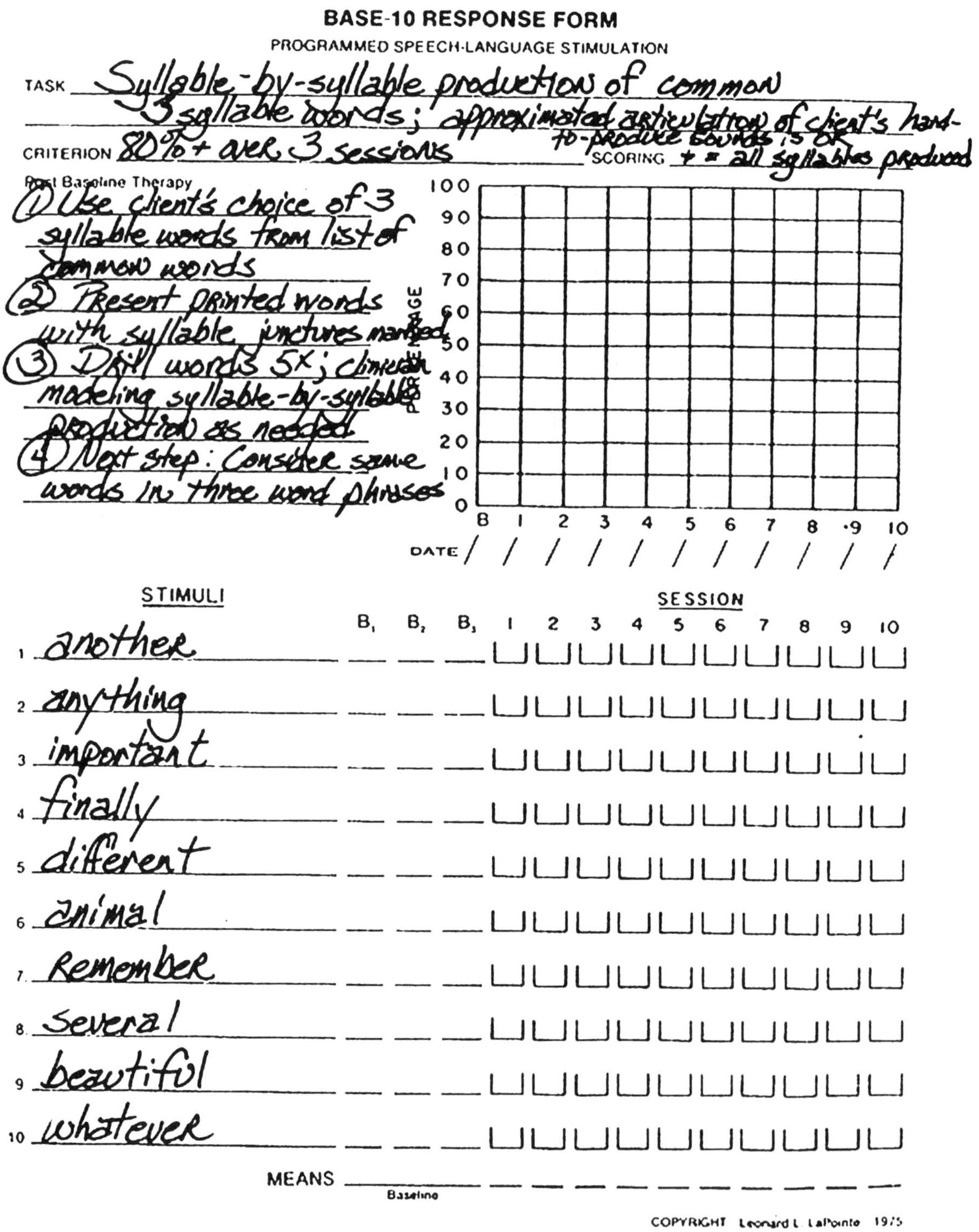

BASE-10 RESPONSE FORM

PROGRAMMED SPEECH-LANGUAGE STIMULATION

TASK: Syllable-by-syllable production of common 3 syllable words; approximated articulation of client's hard-to-produce sounds is OK

CRITERION: 80% + over 3 sessions

SCORING: + = all syllables produced

Post Baseline Therapy

(1) Use client's choice of 3 syllable words from list of common words
(2) Present printed words with syllable junctures marked
(3) Drill words 5X; clinician modeling syllable-by-syllable production as needed
(4) Next step: Consider same words in three word phrases

PERCENTAGE: 100, 90, 80, 70, 60, 50, 40, 30, 20, 10, 0

B 1 2 3 4 5 6 7 8 9 10

DATE / / / / / / / / / / /

STIMULI	B_1	B_2	B_3	1	2	3	4	5	6	7	8	9	10
1 another													
2 anything													
3 important													
4 finally													
5 different													
6 animal													
7 Remember													
8 Several													
9 beautiful													
10 whatever													

MEANS ______ (Baseline)

Figure 10–3. Task: Syllable-by-syllable production of 3-syllable words.

of single syllable words with a smoother, more natural prosody.

Figure 10–4 shows a task developed for a speaker of American English as a second language. On initial testing all speech sounds at the beginning of short words were accurate or fairly approximated; however, he consistently omitted sounds in the word-final position.

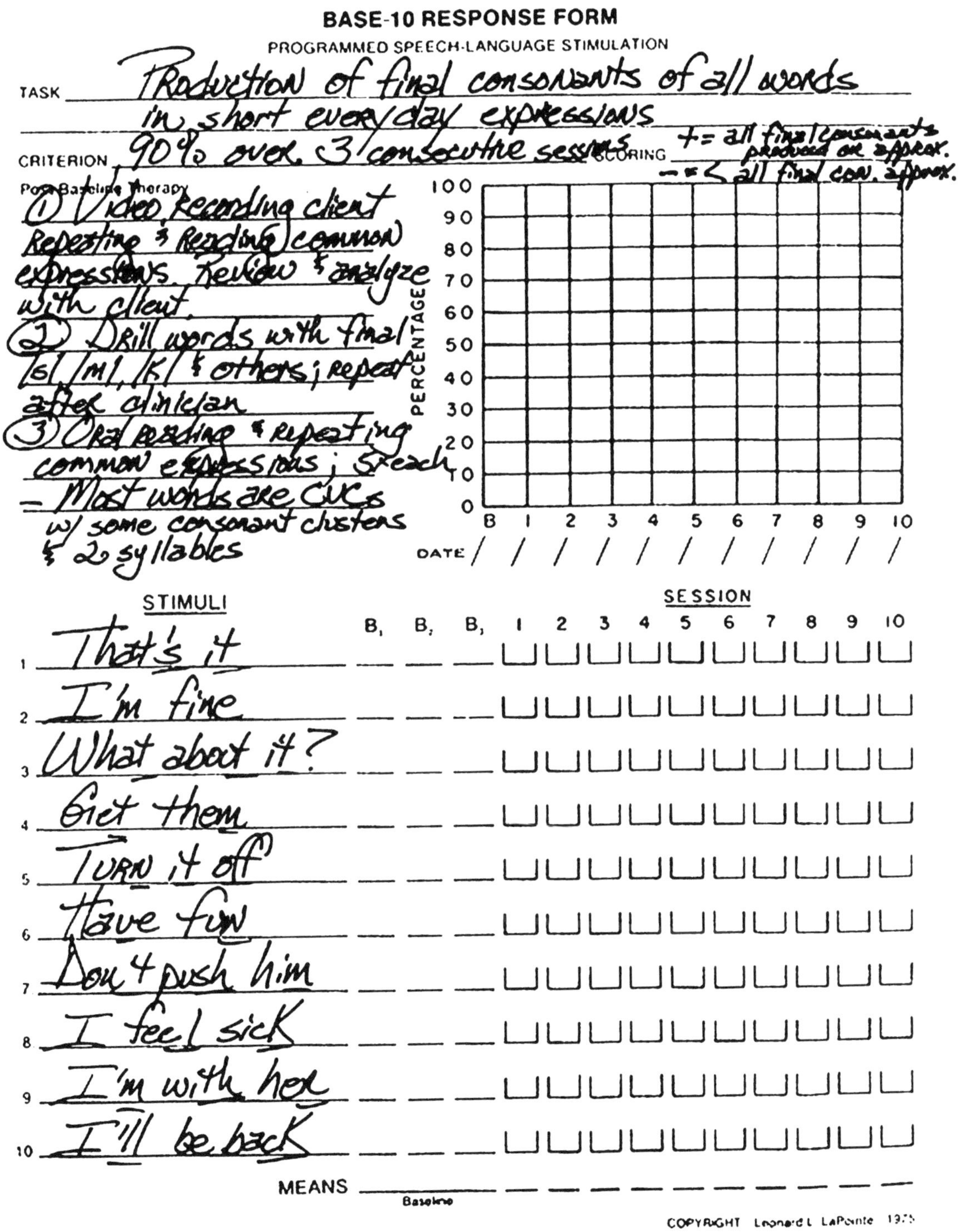

BASE-10 RESPONSE FORM

PROGRAMMED SPEECH-LANGUAGE STIMULATION

TASK: Production of final consonants of all words in short everyday expressions

CRITERION: 90% over 3 consecutive sessions

SCORING: + = all final consonants produced or approx. − = < all final con. approx.

Post-Baseline Therapy: ① Video recording client repeating & reading common expressions. Review & analyze with client. ② Drill words with final /b/ /m/, /k/ & others; repeat after clinician ③ Oral reading & repeating common expressions; 5 each – Most words are CVCs w/ some consonant clusters & 2 syllables

PERCENTAGE: 100, 90, 80, 70, 60, 50, 40, 30, 20, 10, 0

B 1 2 3 4 5 6 7 8 9 10

DATE / / / / / / / / / / /

STIMULI — SESSION: B₁ B₂ B₃ 1 2 3 4 5 6 7 8 9 10

1. That's it
2. I'm fine
3. What about it?
4. Get them
5. Turn it off
6. Have fun
7. Don't push him
8. I feel sick
9. I'm with her
10. I'll be back

MEANS — Baseline

COPYRIGHT Leonard L. LaPointe 1975

Figure 10–4. Task: Production of final consonants.

This was the primary reason his speech was markedly unintelligible in conversation. After some treatment he was able to produce word-final sounds in single CVC words. A possible next step was to address production of all word-final sounds in short, common phrases.

Figure 10–5 displays a task developed for a man who had a traumatic brain injury with

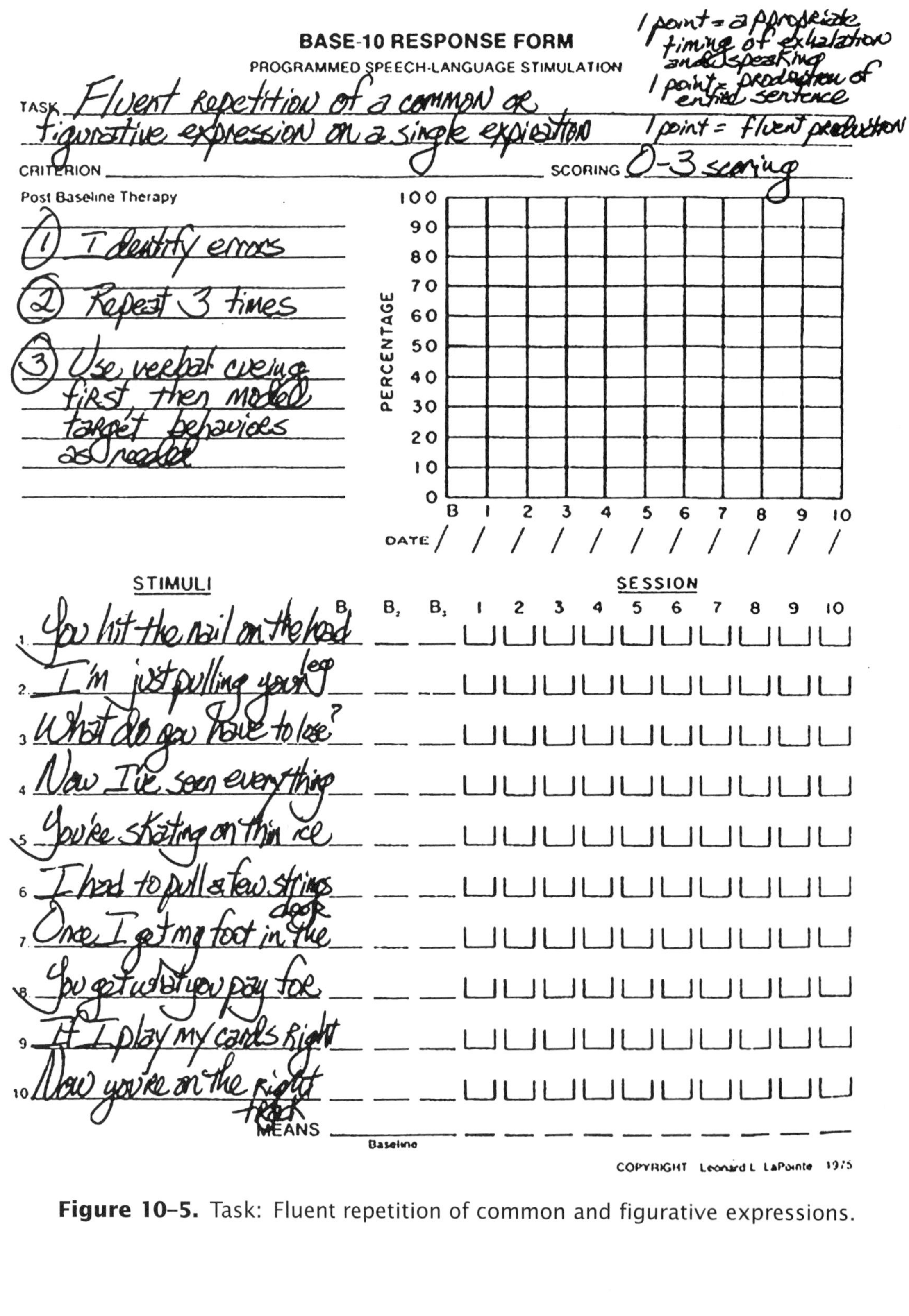

BASE-10 RESPONSE FORM

PROGRAMMED SPEECH-LANGUAGE STIMULATION

TASK Fluent repetition of a common or figurative expression on a single expiration

CRITERION

SCORING 0-3 scoring

1 point = appropriate timing of exhalation and speaking

1 point = production of entire sentence

1 point = fluent production

Post Baseline Therapy

1. Identify errors
2. Repeat 3 times
3. Use verbal cueing first, then model target behaviors as needed

PERCENTAGE 100 90 80 70 60 50 40 30 20 10 0

B 1 2 3 4 5 6 7 8 9 10

DATE / / / / / / / / / / /

STIMULI	B₁	B₂	B₃	1	2	3	4	5	6	7	8	9	10
1. You hit the nail on the head													
2. I'm just pulling your leg													
3. What do you have to lose?													
4. Now I've seen everything													
5. You're skating on thin ice													
6. I had to pull a few strings													
7. Once I get my foot in the door													
8. You get what you pay for													
9. If I play my cards right													
10. Now you're on the right track													
MEANS	Baseline												

Figure 10–5. Task: Fluent repetition of common and figurative expressions.

residual mild cognitive impairment and mixed spastic-ataxic-hypokinetic dysarthria. In addition, he demonstrated moderate dysfluencies characterized by hesitancy and repetition of initial syllables. He was most concerned about the stuttering-like behavior. The timing and coordination of his breathing and speaking efforts were ill synchronized in that he exhaled much or most of his breath before he spoke, resulting in production of only a few words per expiration. Gradually his fluency improved when he focused upon being more fluent. At this point in therapy, a task was developed for him to repeat after the clinician common and figurative expressions of sentence length on a single expiration without dysfluencies. The 0-to-3 scoring system allowed one point each for initiating speech near the beginning of an expiration, completing the expression on one breath, and producing it without hesitation or repetition.

LaPointe (1977, pp. 102-103) described a task for an aphasic person post CVA who demonstrated " . . . unintelligible differentiated jargon, some neologistic jargon, and moderate phonological selection and sequencing impairment" (Figure 10–6). One of the characteristics of the client's speech was substitution of phonemes. LaPointe developed a task for the client to produce sets of rhyming CV and CVC words in which the initial consonants varied in manner of production. The bold vertical lines at Session #4 and Session #5 on the graph indicate when the client was rechecked after 5 months and 11 months had lapsed since Session #3. See LaPointe's original work for additional information about the client, the therapeutic task, and how the specificity built into the Base-10 Response Form and approach to therapy confirmed the subjective impression that the client's speech had improved over time.

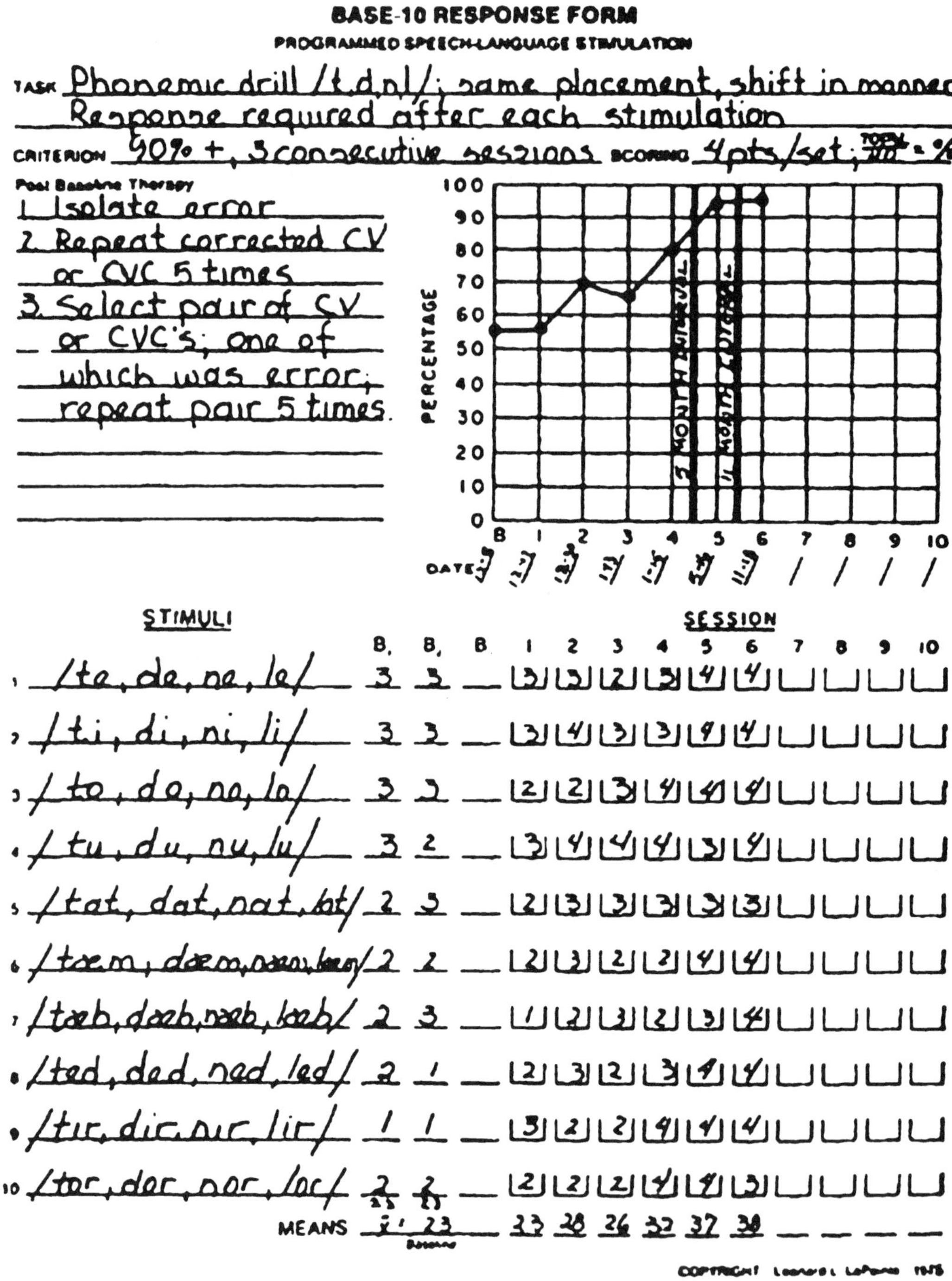

Figure 10–6. Task: Phonemic drill on manner shift. Reprinted with permission from Base-10 Programmed Stimulation: Task Specification, Scoring, and Plotting Performance in Aphasia Therapy by L. L. LaPointe. *Journal of Speech and Hearing Disorders, 42*, 90–105. Copyright 1977 by American Speech-Language-Hearing Association. All rights reserved.

APPENDIX 10-A

Examples of Clinician-Constructed Scoring Systems and Conversion of Base-10 Task Score Sums to Percentages for Graphing

Plus/minus scoring minus = incorrect plus = correct	The total number of correct responses in a column is multiplied by 10 for conversion to a percentage which is entered on the graph for that session. Example: Column total = +4 × 10 = 40%
0- to 2-point scoring Example: 0 = error 1 = approximated response 2 = target response	Scores in a column are added and the total is multiplied by 5 for conversion to percentage. Example: Column total = 14 × 5 = 70%
0- to 3-point scoring Example: 0 = frank error 1 = related, but off-target response 2 = response very close to target 3 = target response	Scores in a column are added and the total is multiplied by 3.3 for conversion to percentage. Example: Column total = 19 × 3.3 = 62%
0- to 4-point scoring Example: See Figure 10-6 illustrating a task requiring a 4-part response, each earning one point	Scores in a column are added and the total is multiplied by 2.5 for conversion to percentage. Example: Column total = 32 × 2.5 = 80%

References

Cooper, R. (1968). The method of meaningful minimal contrasts in functional articulation problems. *Journal of the Speech and Hearing Association of Virginia, 10*, 17-22.

Darley, F. L. (1982). *Aphasia.* Philadelphia: W. B. Saunders.

Duffy, J. R. (2005). *Motor speech disorders: Substrates, differential diagnosis, and management* (2nd ed.). St. Louis, MO: Elsevier-Mosby.

Fairbanks, G. (1960). *Voice and articulation drillbook* (2nd ed.). New York: Harper & Row.

Frattali, C., & Worrall, L. E. (2001). Evidence-based practice: Applying science to the art of clinical care. *Journal of Medical Speech-Language Pathology, 9*, ix-xi.

Kamhi, A. G., & Pollock, K. E. (2005). *Phonological disorders in children: Clinical decision making in assessment and intervention*. Baltimore: Paul H. Brookes.

Kent, R. D. (1976). Models of speech production. In N. Lass (Ed.), *Contemporary issues in experimental phonetics* (pp. 79-104). New York: Academic Press.

LaPointe, L. L. (1977). Base-10 programmed stimulation: Task specification, scoring and plotting performance in aphasia therapy.*Journal of Speech and Hearing Disorders, 42*, 90-105.

LaPointe, L. L. (1985). Aphasia therapy: Some principles and strategies for treatment. In D. F. Johns (Ed.), *Clinical management of neurogenic communicative disorders* (2nd ed., pp. 179-241). Boston: Little, Brown and Company.

LaPointe, L. L. (1991). *Base-10 response form (Revised Manual)*. San Diego, CA: Singular.

Porch, B. E. (1981). *Porch Index of Communicative Ability.* Palo Alto, CA: Consulting Psychologists Press.

Schuell, H., Jenkins, J. J., & Jimenez-Pabon, E. (1964). *Aphasia in adults: Diagnosis, prognosis, and treatment*. New York: Harper & Row.

Van Riper, C., & Irwin, J. (1958). *Voice and articulation*. Englewood Cliffs, NJ: Prentice-Hall.

Vaughn, G. R., & Clark, R. M. (1979). *Speech facilitation: Extraoral and intraoral stimulation technique for improvement of articulation skills.* Springfield, IL: Charles C. Thomas.

Wambaugh, J. L., Duffy, J. R., McNeil, M. R., Robin, D. A., & Rogers, M. A. (2006). Treatment guidelines for acquired apraxia of speech: Treatment descriptions and recommendations. *Journal of Medical Speech-Language Pathology. 14* (2), xxxv-lxvii.

Weiner, F. (1981). Treatment of phonological disability using the method of meaningful minimal contrast: Two case studies. *Journal of Speech and Hearing Disorders, 46*, 97-103.

Wertz, R. T., LaPointe, L. L., & Rosenbek, J. C. (1991). *Apraxia of speech in adults: The disorder and its management.* San Diego, CA: Singular.

Yorkston, K. M., Beukelman, D. R., Strand, E. A., & Bell, K. R. (1999). *Management of motor speech disorders in children and adults* (2nd ed.). Austin, TX: Pro-Ed.

Young, E. H., & Hawk, S. S. (1955). *Moto-kinesthetic speech training.* Palo Alto, CA: Stanford University Press.

Index

G

H

L

P

S

V

W